AF885343

ISBN 978-0-578-76910-3

Any references to historical events, real people, or real places are used fictitiously. Names, characters, and places are products of the author's imagination.

Copyright © 2020 by International Respiratory Infections Society (IRIS)
https://www.irisociety.com/

All rights reserved. This book or any portion thereof may not be reproduced or used in any manner whatsoever without the express written permission of the publisher except for the use of brief quotations in a book review.

Cover design and book design by Kimberley Buckner.

First printing, 2020.

The authors express appreciation for the work of the Immunization Action Coalition (IAC) to enable competent immunization practice. Some of the tools and re-sources developed by IAC are included or referenced throughout the manual, and readers are encouraged to go to the IAC website www.immunize.org to learn more about the vital and growing field of immunization.

Planning and Implementing a Drive-Through Vaccination Process: A Complete How-To Manual

Ruth Carrico, Dawn Balcom,

Kimberley Buckner, Luanne Didelot,

J. Hudson Garrett Jr., Dennis Sullivan

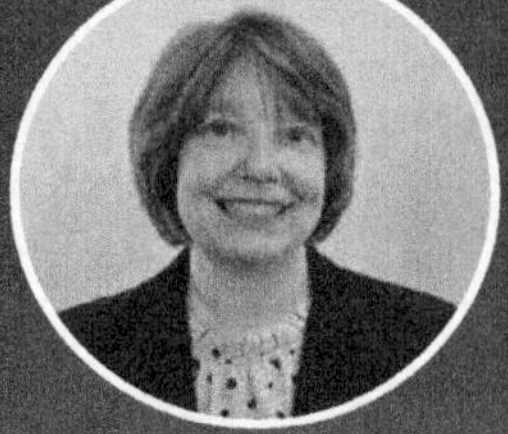

RUTH CARRICO

PhD, DNP, APRN, FNP-C, CIC, FHSEA, FNAP

Professor, Division of Infectious Diseases

Director of Epidemiological Research, Center of Excellence for Research in Infectious Diseases (CERID)

Director, Clinical Research Internship Program

Clinical Director, Vaccine & International Travel Clinic

University of Louisville
School of Medicine
501 E. Broadway, Suite 110
Louisville, KY 40202

Phone: 502.852.6485
Clinic phone: 502.852.6464 Office
fax: 502.852.1420

ruth.carrico@louisville.edu

Ruth Carrico is a Professor and Family Nurse Practitioner with the University of Louisville School Medicine, Division of Infectious Diseases, and director of epidemiological research in the University's Center of Excellence for Research in Infectious Diseases (CERID). Dr. Carrico has received training specific for healthcare epidemiology at the Centers for Disease Control and Prevention (CDC) in conjunction with the Rollins School of Public Health at Emory University in Atlanta and the Society for Healthcare Epidemiology of America (SHEA).

Dr. Carrico is responsible for the clinical and research operations at the University of Louisville Vaccine and International Travel clinic. Her research has been funded by the CDC, HRSA, DHS, and industry.

In 2008, Dr. Carrico was appointed to the National Biosurveillance Subcommittee (NBS) Advisory Committee to the Director, Centers for Disease Control and Prevention, and in 2010 became a SHEA Fellow. In 2011, Dr. Carrico was appointed by Secretary Sebelius, to the Healthcare Infection Control Practices Advisory Committee (HICPAC) for an extended three-year term. In 2012, she was presented with the Carole DeMille Achievement Award by APIC, an honor for an Infection Preventionist. In 2013, Dr. Carrico was appointed to the National Foundation for Infectious Diseases as the Board's Nurse Planner and in 2014 became a Robert Wood Johnson Foundation Executive Nurse Fellow alumna. Dr. Carrico served as the 2016 president of the Certification Board of Infection Control and Epidemiology, Inc. (CBIC), the organization responsible for board certification for infection preventionists worldwide and is now enjoying the role of immediate past president. In 2016, Dr. Carrico co-founded the Infection Prevention Institute a virtual training site focusing on infection prevention education for all partners concerned with preventing infection in any setting. Then, in 2017, the University of Louisville's Journal of Refugee and Global Health was launched, with the first issue released in April of that year. Dr. Carrico serves as the Editor-in-Chief for this new open access journal. In 2018, Dr. Carrico assumed the position of president of the Kentucky Nurses Association and in 2020 was recognized as a Distinguished Fellow in the National Academies of Practice.

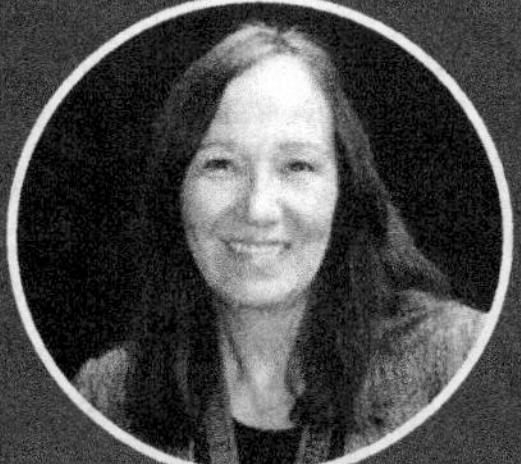

DAWN BALCOM

DNP, MSN, APRN, FNP-C

Family Nurse Practitioner,
Specialist,
Division of Infectious Diseases

Community Engagement Lead,
Center of Excellence for
Research in Infectious Diseases
(CERID)

University of Louisville
School of Medicine
501 E. Broadway, Suite 110
Louisville, KY 40202

Office phone: 502.852.7447
Clinic phone: 502.852.6464
Fax: 502.852.1420
Dawn.balcom@louisville.edu

Dawn Balcom DNP, is a Family Nurse Practitioner with the University of Louisville School of Medicine, Division of Infectious Diseases. Dr. Balcom currently manages the Community Engagement Unit for the division's Center of Excellence for Research in Infectious Diseases, engaging new stakeholders for support in research of emerging infectious diseases and vaccine studies. Dr. Balcom also oversees the division's employee health vaccination program to ensure new researchers and employees joining the division meet and maintain vaccination requirements necessary for continual research in hospitals, outpatient settings, and long-term care facilities. She serves as a mentor to new employees at the University of Louisville Vaccine and International Travel Clinic to ensure development of a comprehensive understanding of workplace proficiencies, knowledge of vaccine preventable diseases, vaccine safety, and reducing vaccine hesitance.

Dr. Balcom has a long interest in emergency medicine and spent 25 years working in the emergency department in large urban hospitals. She obtained her Certification in Emergency Nursing (CEN) and continues to engage emergency medical services into research studies. Dr. Balcom also served at the US Embassy in Singapore providing primary care, travel health consultations, and routine vaccinations to children, adolescents, and adults. She has worked as a primary care provider for the refugee population and has managed multiple large-scale vaccination clinics. She was awarded two service awards while working in Singapore and in 2018 was awarded The Florence Nightingale Award in Nursing.

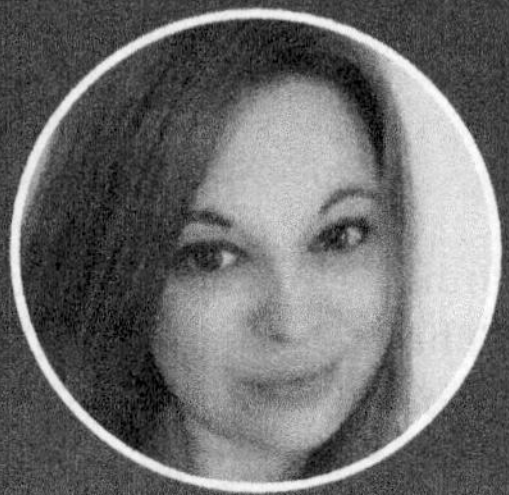

KIMBERLEY BUCKNER

BA

Clinical Research Coordinator,
Division of Infectious Diseases

Education & Training Lead,
Center of Excellence for Research in Infectious Diseases (CERID)

University of Louisville
School of Medicine
501 E. Broadway, Suite 110
Louisville, KY 40202

Phone: 502.852.6464
Office fax: 502.852.1420
Kim.buckner@louisville.edu

Kimberley Buckner is a Clinical Research Coordinator and the Education and Training Lead for the Division of Infectious Diseases Center of Excellence for Research in Infectious Diseases (CERID) at the University of Louisville School of Medicine. She is also a founding officer of the International Respiratory Infections Society. As the managing editor for the launch of both the Journal of Respiratory Infections (JRI) and the Journal of Refugee and Global Health (RGH), open access academic journals, she was integral in developing procedures for publication and indexing.

Kimberley is from Montreal, Canada where she completed her undergraduate degree in Sociology and Psychology from McGill University. Kim brings a perspective and methods of the disciplines of medical sociology and health psychology, both of which have a long history of research into public health issues. After joining the University of Louisville and the Division of Infectious Diseases, Kim helped bring technologies to the research infrastructure in database development and the corresponding clinical research practices. Her unique abilities to engage individuals and groups as part of research and education led her to explore use of web-based training technologies and strategies. The coronavirus pandemic demonstrated the value of her skill sets and through them she worked to bring a model of training and education built upon the approaches used by Project ECHO. She has successfully led the development and launching of the Project ECHO Infection Control series at a time when that subject matter is of critical importance in every area of patient care. This work has formed the basis for the Regional Training Center focused on infection control and operated in collaboration with the University of Louisville Division of Infectious Diseases, CERID, and the Kentucky Department for Public Health.

Kim is currently completing her Master of Professional Studies in Organizational Development and Change from Pennsylvania State University and is putting this knowledge and professional competence in action at the University of Louisville.

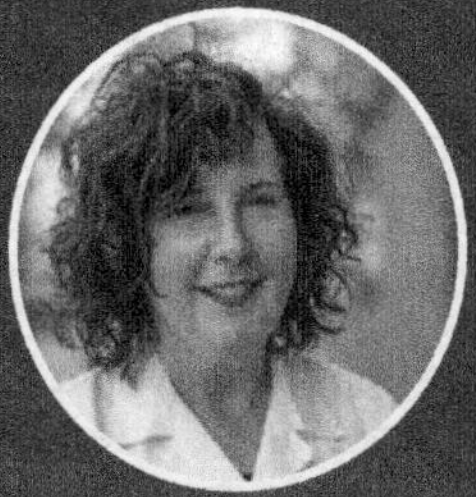

LUANNE DIDELOT

MHA, MSN

Senior Nurse Specialist,
Vaccine & International
Travel Clinic,
Division of Infectious Diseases

University of Louisville
School of Medicine
501 E. Broadway, Suite 110
Louisville, KY 40202

Office phone: 502.852.6436
Clinic phone: 502.852.6464
Fax: 502.852.1420
luanne.didelot@louisville.edu

Luanne Didelot is a Senior Nurse Specialist with the University of Louisville School of Medicine, Division of Infectious Diseases. She is certified by the International Society of Travel Medicine as a Travel Medicine Specialist and assists clients in navigating medical preparation for travel abroad. It is her passion to educate patients on vaccine related illness and provide top flight Travel Medicine services. Experience during her tenure within the Division of Infectious Diseases includes coordinating off-site vaccination clinics serving thousands of refugees annually through two Kentucky resettlement agencies. She also coordinates research activities within the Vaccine and International Travel Clinic and enjoys teaching and training professionals about vaccine related best practice topics.

Her educational background includes degrees from Indiana University including a Master of Health Administration from the School of Public and Environmental Affairs, and Master of Nursing Administration from the IU School of Nursing.

Her many years of nursing experience include hospital administration, managing Primary Care as a Center of Excellence in a large urban tertiary care facility, school nursing for a corporation of over 12,000 students with a diverse population, supervising a large adult diabetic medical-surgical unit, coordinating cardiovascular clinical research trials, and developing a global cardiovascular surgical training program for physicians performing investigational procedures.

Luanne received Indiana University's prestigious President's Award from the I.U. Alumni Association and was recognized as an "Outstanding Alumni" by the I.U. Division of Nursing. She is a Fellow of Greater Louisville Inc's, Health Enterprise Network, and has been an active volunteer performing in leadership roles for the Girl Scouts of Kentuckiana and Boy Scouts of America –Lincoln Heritage Council.

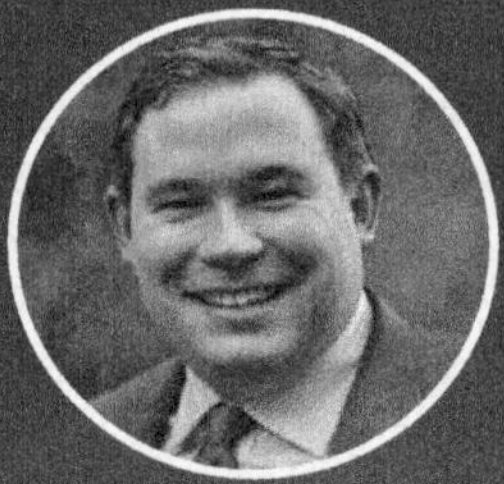

HUDSON GARRETT JR.

PhD, MSN, MPH, MBA, FNP-BC, IP-BC, PLNC, CFER, AS-BC, VA-BC, MSL-BC, CPPS, CPHQ, FACDONA, FAAPM, FNAP

Adjunct Assistant Professor of Medicine, Division of Infectious Diseases

University of Louisville
School of Medicine
Hudson.garrett@louisville.edu

Dr. Hudson Garrett has a faculty appointment as an Adjunct Assistant Professor of Medicine in the Division of Infectious Diseases at the University of Louisville School of Medicine. He also co-founded the nonprofit the Infection Prevention Institute to help shepherd dissemination of best practices of infection prevention and control across the healthcare continuum of care globally. He holds a Graduate Certificate in Infection Prevention and Infection Control from the University of South Florida. He has completed the Johns Hopkins Fellows Program in Hospital Epidemiology and Infection Control. He is also a Fellow in the Academy of National Associations of Directors of Nursing Administration, the American Academy of Project Management, and a Senior Fellow of the Management and Strategy Institute. In 2019, he was inducted as a Distinguished Fellow and Practitioner in the National Academies of Practices. He holds graduate certificates in healthcare leadership from both Cornell and the University of Notre Dame. He is an appointed member of the advisory committee for the Design Thinking in Healthcare Program at Rutgers University. He is a frequent international lecturer in the areas of infectious diseases, healthcare associated infections, outbreak response and prevention and infection prevention and control. He holds Board Certifications in Patient Safety, Healthcare Quality, Vascular Access, Antibiotic Stewardship, Prehospital Emergency Medical Services, Flexible Endoscope Reprocessing, Critical Care, and Infection Prevention and Control in Post-Acute Care.

Dr. Garrett led the development of the first and only core infection prevention and control and antibiotic stewardship certifications and certificate of mastery programs in postacute care settings. He has served on international and national organizational boards in the areas of environmental services, dental infection control, infection control, acute care infection control, post-acute care infection control, and vascular access. He has served on expert panels related to disinfection and sterilization with the United States Food, Centers for Disease Control and Prevention, and Drug Administration and Environmental Protection Agency, most notably serving on the FDA's Panel and Working Group for Flexible Endoscope Reprocessing. Dr. Garrett has lectured in more than 25 countries and given testimony to government and regulatory agencies on a variety of topics related to infectious diseases.

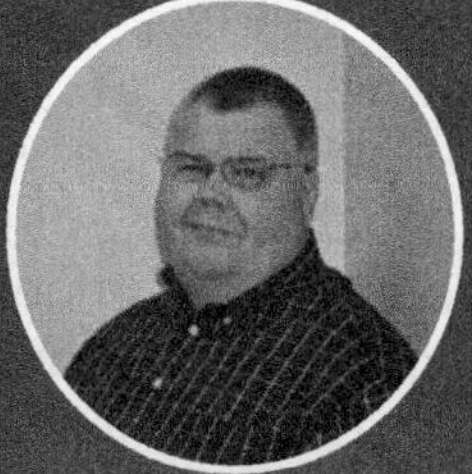

DENNIS SULLIVAN

BA, EMT-P, CHMM, CEM

Adjunct Instructor,
National Center for Bio-Terrorism Response and Training, Academy of Counter-Terrorism Education
Louisiana State University

Contract Instructor Emergency Management Institute, Federal Emergency Management Agency

Department of Homeland Security
918 Eastern Parkway Louisville, KY

Phone: 502.592.1178
dennissullivan@lsu.edu
dennis.sullivan@louisville.edu

Dennis Sullivan is an Adjunct Instructor for the Louisiana State University National Center for Bioterrorism Response and Training/Academy of Counter-Terrorism Education. LSU NCBRT/ACE is a nationally recognized center for emergency preparedness and response training located at Louisiana State University's flagship campus in Baton Rouge, Louisiana. The Center's Instructors provide mobile training to both the national and international emergency response community. Together with stakeholders, NCBRT/ACE influence human safety, security, and resilience in a positive manner. Mr. Sullivan is also a Contract Instructor for the Federal Emergency Management Agency Emergency Management Institute providing mobile training at campuses and other private, state, and federal facilities. In addition, Mr. Sullivan is an instructor specializing in Emergency Management for academic and business campuses, government and private facilities and Integrated Active Shooter Response.

Mr. Sullivan began his career with the Emergency Medical Services (EMS) in Jefferson County (Louisville) as a Paramedic and moved up through the service to the position of Deputy Director for Operations. In that position, he was instrumental in developing the community's Hazardous Materials Response Team. This work led to his becoming a Contract Instructor for the Agency for Toxic Substance and Disease Registry, an agency of the Centers for Disease Control and Prevention.

Upon his retirement from EMS, Mr. Sullivan continued to work as needed as a Paramedic and was certified for a total of 37 years. Following his retirement from Jefferson County EMS, Mr. Sullivan assumed the position as the Assistant Director of Environmental Health and Safety at the University of Louisville where he also served as the University's Emergency Manager. During his tenure at the University, Mr. Sullivan obtain his certifications as an Emergency Manager (international Association of Emergency Managers, state certification as an Emergency Manager and a Certified Hazardous Materials Manager (Alliance of Hazardous Materials Professionals).

During his 26 years at the university, he worked with Dr. Ruth Carrico to plan and implement the largest mass immunization event held in the United States which has since become a planning tool for others.

Preface

Things were relatively quiet in late 2019 as we were reading about a new respiratory illness identified in China. Little did we realize that we were experiencing the front end of a new pandemic, an event we forecast as occurring only once in a lifetime. As this novel virus moved around the globe, we began to realize the potential need to immunize the 7 billion inhabitants on the planet. Also, the timing of this pandemic was destined to coincide with the annual emergence of influenza and potentially represent a twin epidemic that could co-exist for years to come. Planning for immunization was immediately challenged due to the entire population having to distance from each other socially, as well as the need to provide vaccines to individuals being in isolation due to suspected COVID-19 illness or quarantine due to exposure. Social distancing measures meant that traditional ways of accessing vaccine in provider offices, pharmacies, workplaces, and schools would be complicated. The use of drive-through vaccination procedures gained renewed interest, and the ability for any group or community to prepare and implement rapidly has emerged as a targeted capability.

This book represents more than twenty-five years of experience with drive-through and mass immunization approaches. It represents the only contemporary and comprehensive summary of information that serves as a guide for groups of communities interested in planning and implementing a drive-through immunization event. Many have worked to plan and implement drive-through COVID-19 testing clinics, and you will find that planning elements are similar. This book should provide added confidence that drive-through immunization events can be conducted safely and efficiently if there is proper attention devoted to the planning phase. Ensuring that the event location is suitable, staff are trained and competent, vaccines are protected, and patients are engaged and informed are critical for safety and community support.

This book contains chapters devoted to the various components of planning and implementing a drive-through vaccination event. Each chapter includes a narrative review of the topic followed by the slides used in presenting that topic as part of a webinar series conducted in July-August 2020. Links are included that will take the reader to a recording of each webinar. Tools and resources relevant to the topic are also provided in each chapter. We expect that readers will use this information to benefit their communities and in support of a vaccination process built upon confident and competent practice.

Ruth Carrico

Ruth Carrico PhD DNP FNP-C

TABLE OF CONTENTS

Chapter 6: Patient Education, Documentation, and Vaccine Information Systems

Chapter 7: Emergency Response in a Drive-Through Vaccination Event

Introduction

When considering the opportunities for immunization, the traditional approach of office or pharmacy locations likely comes immediately to mind. However, experiences have shown that vaccines administered in alternative settings can address community and society needs, including added convenience and heightened infection control. Drive-through vaccination was first documented in the fall of 1994 in Louisville, Kentucky, as part of community outreach and influenza immunization. The goal of that program was to provide access to the influenza vaccine by those whose access may be limited by mobility, time, and location accessibility and availability. During that first drive-through, approximately 800 Louisvillians were vaccinated, and the population vaccinated spanned all ages from infants to the frail elderly. That same year, as the drive-through was being planned, colleagues from the Visiting Nurses Association were planning the provision of influenza vaccine at local grocery stores. The two groups planning these independent, yet related events worked side by side to consider patient safety, infection control, and community acceptance. At that time, there was concern that the community would not view immunization favorably when it occurred outside the provider office and that there would be safety concerns associated with immunization in cars and grocery stores. However, history has shown these concerns to be unfounded, and drive-through vaccination programs have been conducted across the United States and the world. The procedures used for drive-through events have informed public health approaches and the basis for mass community immunization. Further, immunization has continued to be provided in grocery stores through pharmacies and associated retail clinics. It is reasonable to consider that implementation of that first drive-through vaccination event in 1994 prompted a revolution as to how immunization can be delivered and how the provision of vaccines in non-traditional ways can support routine immunization for children, adolescents, and adults.

Following the first drive-through in 1994, hospitals and health departments across the US began to contact the team at the University of Louisville Hospital (now UofL Health) requesting information so they could plan and conduct similar events. Written procedures were shared and refined, and in 2002, the first 'how-to' book was published that provided step-by-step instructions for those interested in developing and scaling a drive-through for an individual office or community needs, based upon a mass immunization model. The approach was also used as public health departments were developing emergency response plans as part of bio-terrorism preparedness and response planning. Point of Dispensing (POD) plans incorporated walk-up and drive-through components, and POD drive-through events were used to train and exercise medical reserve corps units across the US, often as part of the Cities Readiness Initiative.

In 2009, national public health was confronted with the need to address the H1N1 influenza pandemic quickly. In Louisville, Kentucky, the local public health department had implemented the drive-through approach for emergency planning, as had the University of Louisville. The two worked together to ramp up a large-scale mass immunization event at the university's football stadium. Industrial engineers from the University of Louisville Speed School of Engineering were engaged to help simulate the processes to enable efficiency and safety. Almost 20,000 doses of vaccine were made available for the drive-through, and all were administered in less than 18 hours. At that time, the event was reportedly the largest such event to have occurred in the US or elsewhere. No errors were identified, and no adverse events were reported.

Following that successful demonstration of mass immunization, in 2010, the National Association of County and City Health Officials (NACCHO) formally embraced the processes. They published a guide for the use of drive-through for point of dispensing in the event of a public health emergency or mass immunization needs building upon the Louisville H1H1 immunization event. In that same year, NACCHO also worked with the National Association of School Nurses (NASN) to use this success in support of stimulating discussion regarding school located vaccination (SLV) clinics. In 2011, the Centers for Disease Control and Prevention (CDC) funded an emergency countermeasures project that involved using drive-through as a demonstration for engaging new workforce supports that could be used for an emergency response to public health needs. This project demonstrated the ability to engage, train, and deploy student nurses quickly as a competent new and continuously available workforce that could be relied upon in emergency situations. The demonstration event was held in the summer heat of July 2011 and was named Operation Popsicle. Influenza vaccines were not yet available for administration that flu season, so Popsicles were used as the vaccine surrogate. Students demonstrated the ability to engage with the patient, select the correct Popsicle "vaccine" and dose (single Popsicle or a double), provide patient education, and administer the Popsicle using a napkin as the surrogate Band-Aid. Training elements were aligned with the curriculum essentials, further demonstrating the ability to incorporate the fundamentals of vaccine, vaccine administration, safety, patient education, and documentation into the healthcare academic programs.

Since that time, drive-through immunization has become a relative staple in communities for routine immunization for the full population spectrum as well as public health planning and regularly engages students in the health and public health sciences.

In early 2020, the SARS-CoV-2 pandemic prompted a renewed interest in drive-through immunization. Social distancing and the need to enable various isolation and quarantine approaches formed the basis for a new conversation regarding the drive-through process. This method of mass vaccination could allow large numbers of individuals to seek vaccination while practicing social distancing in their car, presumably with individuals from their "bubble." The team of healthcare providers and planners that had developed the first event in 1994 and subsequent others came together to provide a series of webinars outlining the steps in a drive-through immunization process that could be used during the 2020-2021 influenza season and as preparation and practice for COVID-19 vaccination.

This e-book contains the basic elements needed for drive-through immunization planning, implementation, and evaluation and represents a complete how-to manual. Chapters are organized to take the reader from the initial planning through staff training, management, and handling of vaccines, patient education and documentation, emergency response, and right-sizing the event to meet community needs. Each chapter contains an overview of that element of the drive-through planning and implementation process, PowerPoint slides from presentations that occured July-August 2020, and some tools and resources that are considered by the authors to represent best practices. Information that enables the readers to access the video recording of each session is also provided as well as additional web links for larger resource documents.

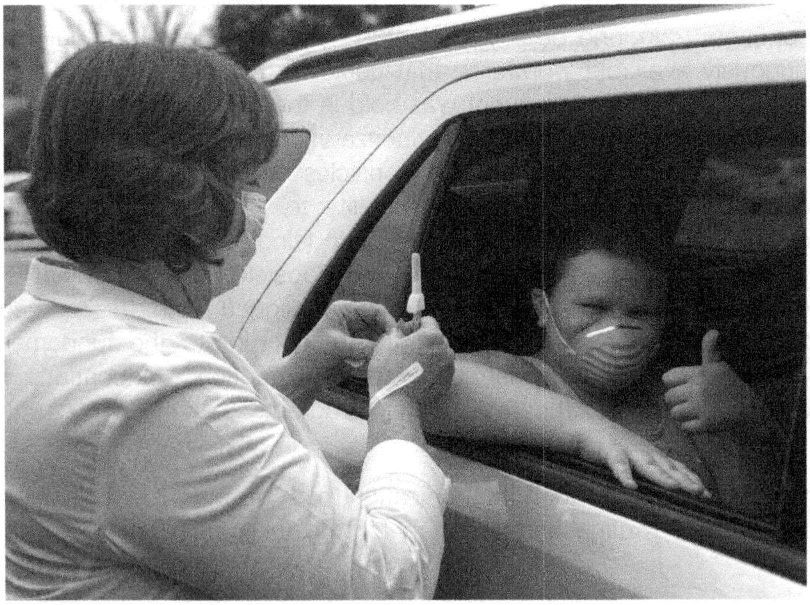

CHAPTER 1

DRIVE-THROUGH VACCINATION: CLINIC SETUP AND LOGISTICS

SAMPLE JOB ACTION SHEET

VISUAL DEPICTION OF DRIVE-THROUGH PROCESS

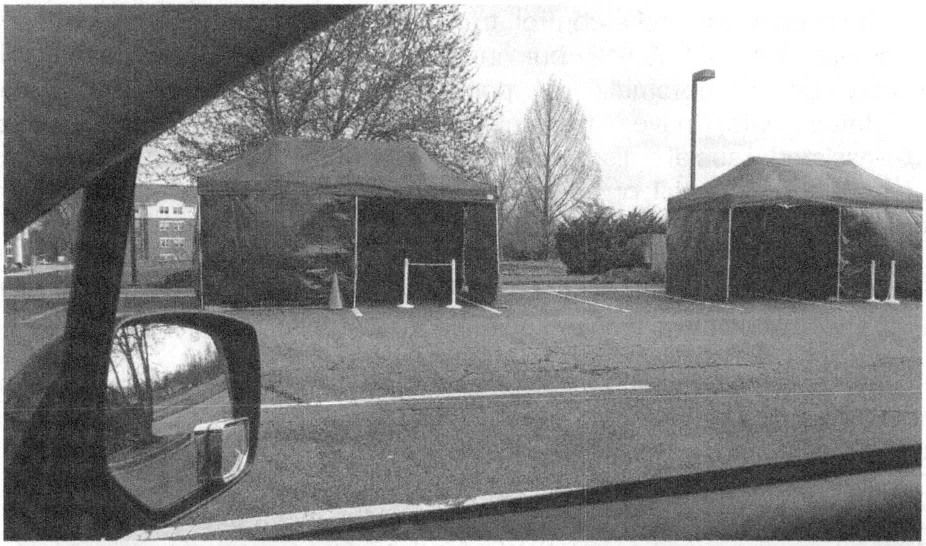

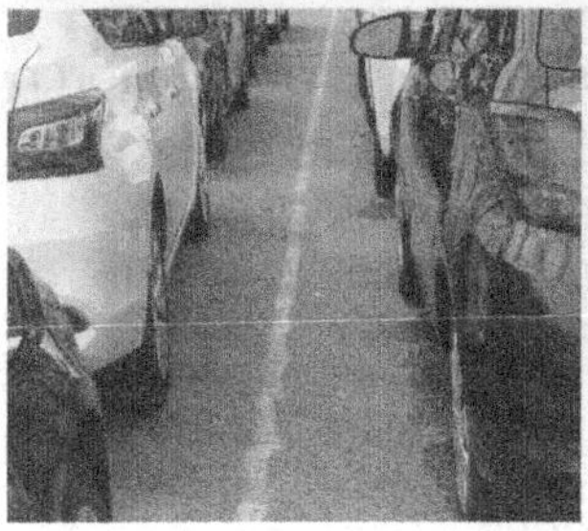

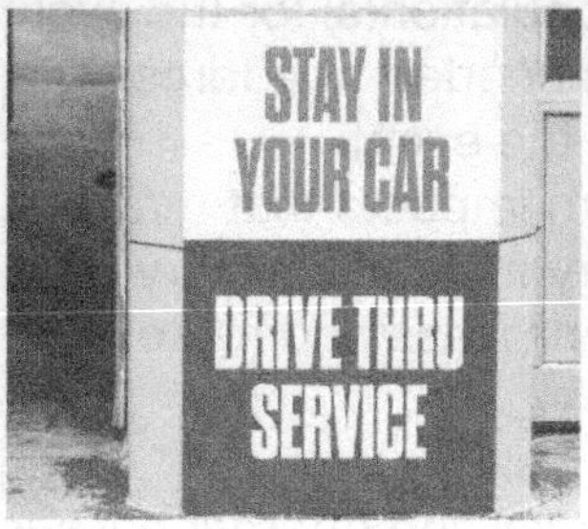

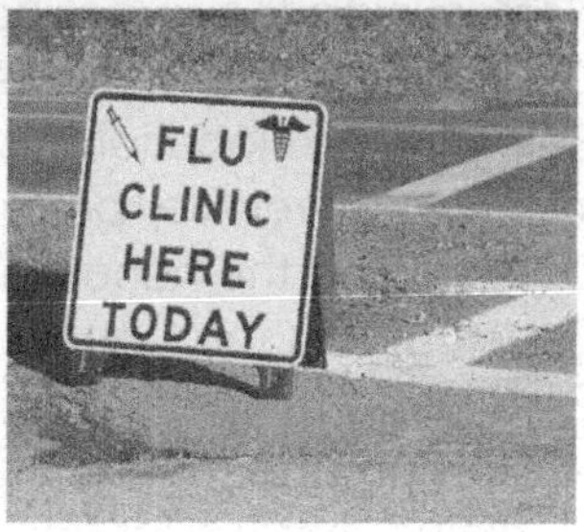

Dennis Sullivan BA, EMT-P, CHMM, CEM, Ruth Carrico PhD DNP FNP-C

Planning for a drive-through immunization event begins with reasons why and how such an approach can contribute to the provision and acceptance of immunization in the population. Historically, drive-through vaccination has focused primarily on influenza immunization during flu season—use of drive-through offered opportunities for those experiencing mobility issues, including the disabled and the elderly. If recipients of the vaccine could stay in their car, this prevented inconveniences of parking and entering the provider office or pharmacy. Drive-through also offers the ability for those fearful of vaccination to use a method that enables them to remain in control. For example, someone afraid of vaccination maintains control when they approach the drive-through event, and if they change their mind, they can always stay in the car and drive away. As we consider the use of a drive-through during the time of COVID-19, the use of this method as a means of maintaining social distancing offers a significant public health benefit while still allowing for immunization across the population. Vehicle social distancing can help control transmission from those who may be symptomatic with COVID-19 but in need of influenza vaccination. Those who may be asymptomatic or per-symptomatic and are unaware of that status will have transmission opportunities minimized through vehicle-assisted social distancing drive-through vaccination. Those without a car have the potential of being included by others in their family or friend "bubble" who have a car or by taking advantage of other ride sharing such as that provided by Uber or Lyft. City planners can also use drive-through with public transportation using city buses as the vehicle and including a drive-through vaccination clinic location as a planned stop.

The key to implementing a drive-through event begins with a solid planning foundation. Elements essential in planning for clinic or event logistics include the following:

- Convening of a planning team
- Conceptualizing the scope of the event and the event plan
- Determining the target population(s) for the event
- Determining the vaccines needed to address the scope and population needs
- Selecting the location for the event
- Identifying weather pattern impacts that may influence the event
- Determining the necessary multidisciplinary staffing
- Developing a throughout process and route
- Simulating the process
- Assessing and managing risk
- Outlining metrics for financial and operational success
- Convening of a planning team

The planning team should consist of some specific areas of expertise, including someone responsible for leading the team and members able to address logistics, safety, compliance, documentation, staffing, infection control, and finance. The team leader should have insight into the entire process and be able to convene a team able to work together collaboratively. At the same time, be able to bring forward dissenting opinions and work together toward a goal-based resolution. The team member responsible for logistics should have the ability to envision the drive-through process and organize an operational approach to meet the drive-through needs. The safety team member is responsible for anticipating and planning for strategies to ensure safety for the vaccine recipients as well as members of the vaccine event team. They should have knowledge of the vaccination process as well as the throughput procedures. The compliance team member should be aware of regulations, standards, and best practices regarding the drive-through process and vaccine administration. The team member responsible for documentation should be focused on documentation of the event stages as well as documentation of the vaccination process. Someone should lead staffing planning with knowledge of vaccines and the vaccination process. This person must have a background in healthcare as a means of ensuring safe practices and appropriate handling of the vaccine. Infection control is a critical element in the drive-through vaccination process so that members of the team should have a healthcare background inclusive of patient care and infection control basic practices. The team member responsible for finance should have experience in managing and monitoring costs and insurance submission and payment. It is essential to recognize that the skill sets needed by this team can be obtained through collaboration between healthcare setting personnel and public health.

The team should begin meeting as soon as the drive-through project is considered and should continue throughout the planning and implementation of the event, as well as through the development of all after-event reports, including a summary finance and safety report.

Conceptualizing the scope of the event and the event plan

The drive-through event should have an articulated area of focus that includes proposed size (e.g., a single office setting, multi-practice collaboration, community-wide event), target populations, types of vaccine(s) to be provided, methods of payment (e.g., insurance, out of pocket payment using cash or credit card [which ones], spending accounts, a combination of methods, potential dates of the event, and potential locations. These considerations will help guide the determination of key partners that can help add to, alter, or achieve the goals of the event.

Determining the target population(s) for the event

The drive-through event planning should determine the target populations at the time of initial planning. This planning is not limited to identifying the ages of individuals that will be vaccinated but must also include the type of vaccines that will be provided. For influenza, this includes considering vaccines for infants as well as those with severe egg allergy and those with faltering immune systems. If the vaccination process includes other vaccines in addition to influenza, the population may extend to those who have already received an influenza vaccine but may need another immunization as part of a "catch-up" or community intervention. A contemporary example may include someone who needs both an influenza vaccine and a COVID-19 vaccine, or only one of those if both are made available. Care must also be taken to ensure that there is the consideration of the entire population in need of vaccination and address the social determinants of health and other disparities that may require additional focus to ensure vaccine and vaccination access.

Determining the vaccines needed to address the scope and population needs

When conducting a drive-through event during the influenza season, the event planners should consider which influenza vaccines are to be made available. This may include considering a full spectrum of injectable vaccines as well as the intranasal vaccine. Whatever is anticipated to address the needs of the targeted populations as well as promote vaccination acceptance should be included in the determination of vaccines to be provided. Overarching questions include whether or not the event will be confined to one vaccine group (e.g., influenza alone) or include other vaccines of need within the population. When considering the vaccines, it is crucial to consider the handling necessities of those vaccines. For example, influenza vaccines require refrigeration, whereas other vaccines such as Varicella require that they are maintained in a frozen state until immediately before administration. Although the CDC Advisory Committee on Immunization Practices (ACIP) does not indicate preferences for vaccines (e.g., whether individuals 65 or older should receive a high dose or adjuvanted vaccine instead of the standard influenza vaccine), it is beneficial to have someone with knowledge regarding vaccines and current research findings to guide these decisions.

Determining the necessary multidisciplinary staffing

Key staff groups include those responsible for venue setup, greeters, those responsible for consent forms or patient identification, vaccinators, patient educators, cashiers/insurance verifiers, security, vaccine monitors, supply runners, waste handlers, communications, and those responsible for venue tear-down. The setup team should be able to manage tents, electricity hookups, signage, and cones. Greeters should be able to meet the cars are they arrive and give initial directions and a brief overview of the process. Those providing consent forms or checking patient identification should be able to answer questions and provide all needed items such as any paperwork that needs to be completed and writing pens if needed. They should verify that children are with their parent(s) or an individual able to provide consent for their vaccination. Vaccinators must be individuals who have received specific training regarding vaccines, patient assessment, contraindications, administration techniques, and general patient interaction. They should have had training that also requires a demonstration of competence. Additional information regarding this in-depth personnel training is included in subsequent chapters in this book. Patient educators should be available to address questions about the vaccine and the illness(es) targeted by the vaccine(s) before receipt of the vaccine and afterward. Those responsible for financial transactions or insurance verification should know those procedures. They should have change available if the use of cash is anticipated. If credit or debit cards are used, there should be a portable credit card machines readily available, so personnel do not need to leave the immediate area. If cash transactions are anticipated, this personnel should be stationed close to security personnel. Cash should be moved from the site regularly, and processes, such as wearing of cash belts or pockets, should be used to keep cash out of the general view of the public. Sufficient cash denominations should be available to provide change, as needed. This should prompt a discussion regarding vaccination charges, so the need for change is minimized (e.g., avoiding a charge that requires change in dollar bills). Individuals must be assigned responsibility for checking vaccine condition temperatures every hour. Runners, or those responsible for monitoring and ensuring supplies are readily available, must be designated and must be aware of supply needs so they can provide adequate supply levels and placement for efficient access. Waste handlers help remove regular trash and have red bags available in the event regulated waste needs removal.

Regulated waste should be the exception, but there should be a red bag available in case it is needed. An individual responsible for ensuring communication must also be designated. This person monitors the availability of cell service in the event there is need to call for additional supplies or vaccines, first responders, or other assistance. Each of these personnel should have written responsibilities. This helps enable training, ensure knowledge regarding expectations, build accountability, and enable performance metrics. An example of a job action sheet outlining responsibilities is included in the resource section of this chapter.

Developing a throughout process and route

Ensuring an efficient entry, vaccination, and exist process is vital for resource stewardship as well as patient safety. When determining the location for the drive-through, the leadership team should map the entire process, including the routes of entry and exit, as well as approximate locations for the various personnel and supplies. This helps ensure that all steps in the vaccination process have been considered and planned for, and the visual tool enables efficient training for all personnel. An example of a venue plan is included in the resource section of this chapter.

Simulating the process

A final step in preparing for the drive-through involves a dynamic simulation. For this portion of the planning operation, an actual dry run should occur. This enables planners to identify areas that may represent a "choke-hold" in the process. It also helps recognize the impact of increased traffic on the surrounding area. Simulation can facilitate needed changes in the process before the event when it may be challenging to make those required alternations.

Assessing and managing risk

Simulating the process can enable recognition of situations that may pose a safety risk. Risks must be identified, so a strategy to mitigate the impact can be implemented. For example, a vaccine reaction is a risk, although a rare event. Emergency procedures should be planned and exercised, and an ability to communicate directly to first responders should be included in the simulation to reduce the safety risks. Programming of emergency numbers into cell phones is another example of risk mitigation.

Under normal circumstances, personal protective equipment needs are limited. However, when considering a drive-through vaccination event when COVID-19 is a risk, additional planning and risk mitigation is needed. An example involves the availability, use, and disposal of personal protective equipment. An entire chapter of this book is devoted to infection control, and more information will be provided. However, one of the planning members must be assigned to address personal protective equipment if needed to ensure training and supply availability, as well as management of the additional waste generated when these items are widely needed and used.

Outlining metrics for financial and operational success

Evaluation of any project begins at the time of project planning. Essential aspects of the project should have a corresponding evaluative metric that can be clearly described to personnel and measured for improvement and reporting purposes. Examples of metrics include the following:

- Accuracy of consent forms (# of forms with error(s)/total # of forms)
- Types of consent form errors (e.g., legibility, completion rate, patient signature)
- Vaccination errors (#incorrect vaccine/ total # doses of that vaccine that should have been administered)
- Patients reporting adverse events
- Payment for vaccination by payment type

A complete financial report is essential to capture the entire history and outcomes of the event. A template for the report developed at the time of the event concept enables an evolving picture of the event that captures all aspects for financial and operational review purposes.

In summary, a strong leadership team consisting of many or a few must be able to conceptualize and address the entire vaccination process so they can ensure team member share the skill sets and areas of needed expertise for a safe, efficient, and effective event. Lack of planning may result in patient or personnel harm, so investing in the time and planning resources provide the best opportunities for ideal outcomes.

When considering how to plan and implement a drive-through vaccination event, focused effort is necessary to ensure you have sufficient numbers of personnel who are each competent to perform their roles and job responsibilities. This makes determining the clinic flow, the staffing needed to complete the work, and the training of those staff in three primary areas of concentration as you prepare for the event.

Sample Job Action Sheet

Instructions for Obtaining Consent at the

Drive-Thru Flu H1N1 Immunization Program

- Always watch out for cars, especially when walking between them.
- Consent forms are on pads, and we will have plenty of pens.
- Give every person receiving a vaccine a pad of consent forms and a pen, if they need one.
- A consent form must be completed for every person who will be receiving the vaccine. Feel free to tear the pads apart and provide a small stack for a firm writing surface
- Provide a copy of the Vaccine Information Sheets (VIS) and place it on the dashboard of each car.
- Leave the consent form and pen with them so they can complete it while they move forward toward the vaccination tent.
- Instruct them to move forward with traffic, and nurses will come to the car at the tent site to administer the vaccine.
- If individuals have questions about any of the vaccines, ask them to roll down their window, and we will have individuals available to answer their questions. Do not delay their movement forward.
- Contraindications for immunization include:
  - People who have a severe allergy (rash or trouble breathing) to chicken eggs (not to feathers or dander and not a gastrointestinal response to eggs).
  - People who have had a severe reaction to influenza vaccination.
  - People who developed Guillain-Barré syndrome (GBS) after receiving the influenza vaccine in the past.
  - Children younger than six months of age (influenza vaccine is not approved for this age group), and
  - People who have a moderate-to-severe illness with a fever of at least 100.4^0F. They should wait until they are improving to be vaccinated.

- If you identify language as a potential barrier to understanding, please direct them toward the far right-hand lane so they can go into the walk-up tent instead of the drive-through. If you detect any special needs that concern you about the ability of the individual to utilize the drive-through process, direct them toward the walk-up tent instead.
- Individuals who have been on Tami-flu or are currently taking Tami-flu can have the injectable vaccine.

Visual Depiction of Drive-Through Process

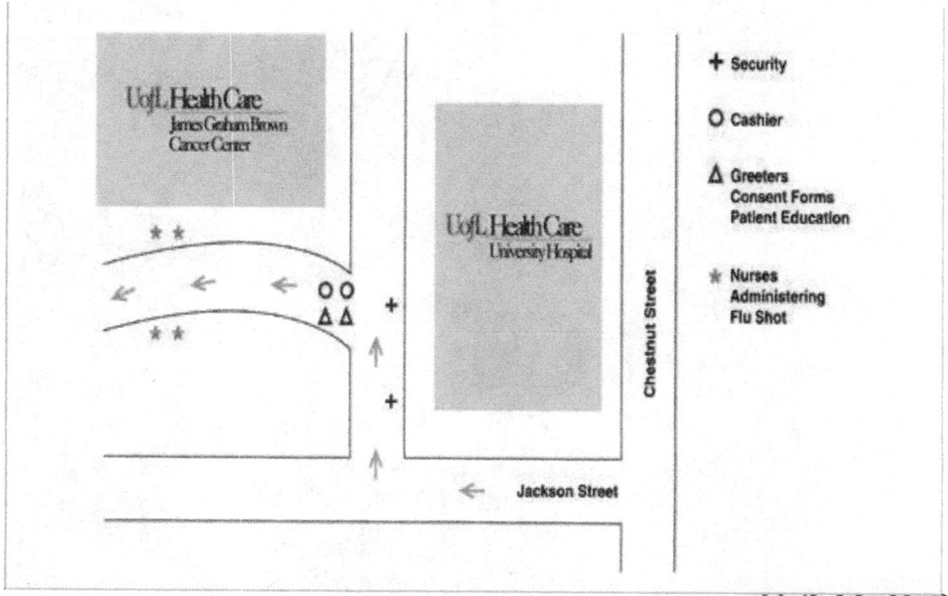

UofL Health Care
University Hospital

CHAPTER 2

DRIVE-THROUGH VACCINATION: CLINIC STAFF AND TRAINING

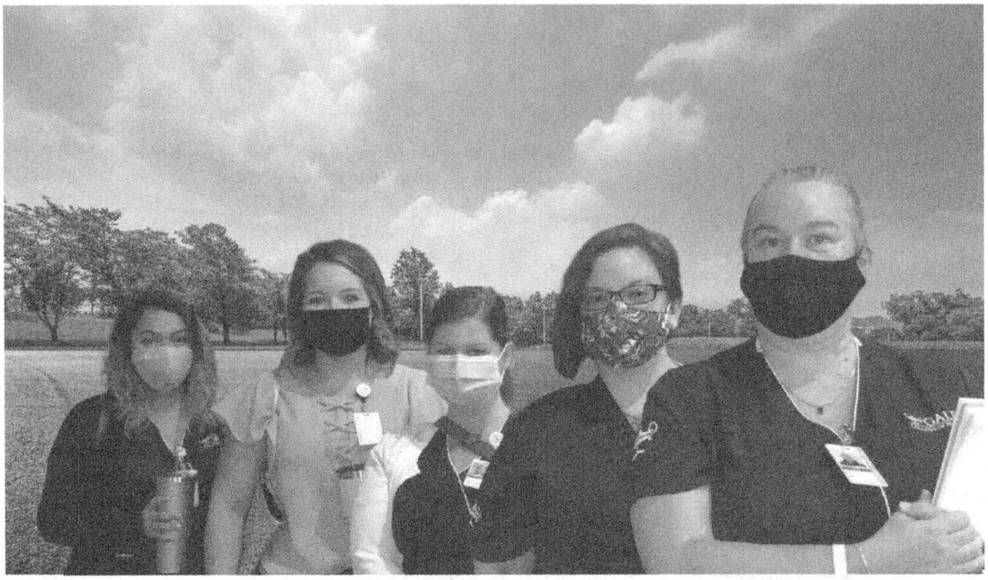

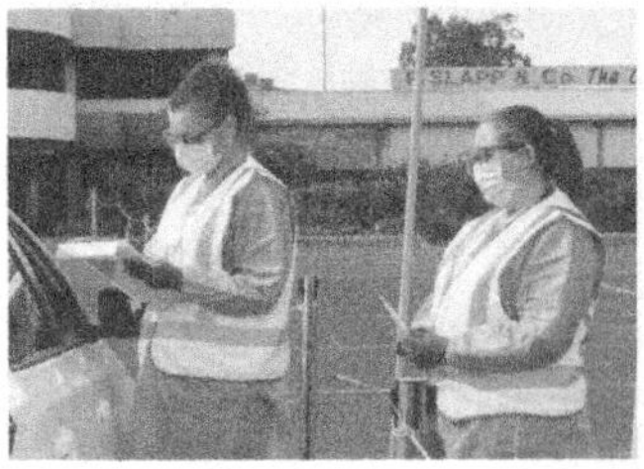

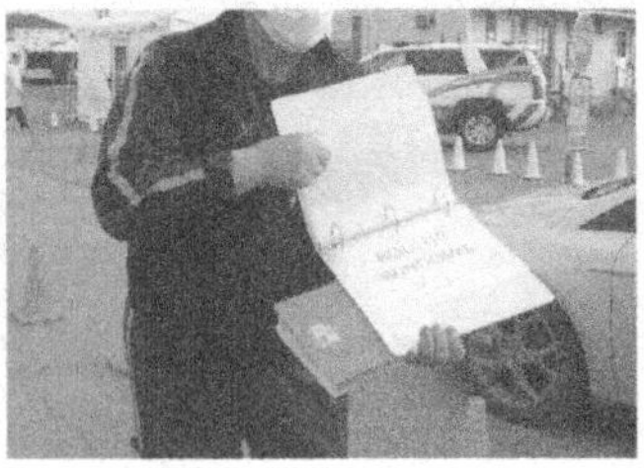

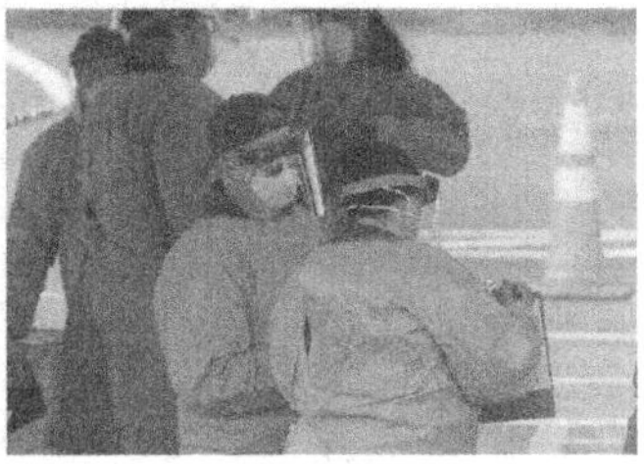

Luanne Didelot MHA MSN, Ruth Carrico PhD DNP FNP-C

When considering how to plan and implement a drive-through vaccination event, focused effort is necessary to ensure you have sufficient numbers of personnel who are each competent to perform their roles and job responsibilities. This makes determining the clinic flow, the staffing needed to complete the work, and the training of those staff in three primary areas of concentration as you prepare for the event.

Clinic Flow

The rst chapter of this book focused on the logistics involved in planning a drive-through vaccination event and outlined the management and oversight structure, including the role of the Team Leader. This team leader should remain separate from the sta ng designated for the various stations as their role is oversight of the entire process. The leadership team, reviewed in another chapter, outlined the core responsibilities for general management of the drive-through operation. This chapter will focus on sta ng and training to safely administer and document vaccination.

Determining the size of the event and the size of the population expected to participate in the event will drive the determination of clinic ow, and ultimately, the sta ng needed to accomplish the vaccination objectives. There will be several "stations" for a vaccination drive-through: 1) point of entry; 2) data or information collection from the vaccine recipient; 3) payment for the vaccine; 4) receipt of the vaccine; 5) education and follow-up, and 6) waiting area and exit. In a smaller-scale event, you may have personnel sta ng more than one of those stations. In larger-scale events, you will likely need multiple personnel for each station and additional personnel that can oat or "run" between stations. Determining how the arriving vehicle will move through the drive-through event will help identify appropriate locations for each station, the amount of space needed between stations, and the course the vehicle will take from arrival to departure from the event site. Simulating the vehicle pathway process is benefi ial for evaluating the ow of vehicles and where to best establish the stations for ease of throughput and accomplishment of the activities necessary at each station. Once your clinic ow has been determined, you are ready to begin working on sta ng needs and planning.

Staffing

When determining the process for assembling a team to perform a large- or small-scale event, it is essential to put aside personality types. The focus should be on how to go about getting the job done! Those with experience can tell you, and it is about putting the right people in the right positions and training them sufficiently. The areas of responsibility for a drive-through event include: 1) greeter; 2) consent and documentation; 3) vaccinator; 4) finance; 5) patient educator; 6) vaccine monitor; 7) supply monitor; 8) infection control monitor; and 9) traffic management. Not each of these roles will be assigned to a particular station. Instead, the roles may have responsibilities that cross stations or are part of the organizational structure and operation of the drive-through.

A greeter will be the first person an arriving vaccine recipient will see, and they should quickly direct them to enter a queue. The number of lines for vaccination will depend on how many people are expected to receive the vaccine(s) and how many personnel can administer the vaccine(s). It is helpful to assign each area of responsibility specific tasks that are all within their ability to perform. This enables the monitoring of performance and rapid correction. The greeter should be assigned three primary responsibilities: 1) greet each arriving car and direct them to the queue; 2) provide a VIS for each vaccine to be administered, placing it on the dashboard of the vehicle; and 3) remind all persons in that vehicle to check and make sure their seatbelt is secure as they move forward. Greeters will be able to direct individuals forward into multiple lines if there is more than one line. Their function is also designed to make the vaccine recipients less anxious, so friendly interaction is essential. Federal law requires that a VIS be made available to the vaccine recipient before the administration of a vaccine. Your clinic process may have already made the VIS available through another route (e.g., electronically). Placing a copy in the vehicle may help refresh the vaccine recipient's memory regarding questions. Color-coding and laminating the VIS can help reuse documents while enabling disinfection. If only inactivated flu vaccine is provided, then only one VIS is needed. Lastly, greeters help promote safety, so reminders about seat belts or pointing attention to signage that may have additional directions helps with the transition to the next station (e.g., prepare to roll up sleeve, have your identification handy, have preprinted consent forms accessible).

The individual responsible for consent documentation should be the next person seen in the queue. This is often the most time-consuming process if vaccine recipients are to each complete a type of consent or documentation form. This documentation is essential, so there is a record of all patients vaccinated in the drive-through event with the ability to contact them if needed. A short paper form can help gather information regarding vaccine contraindication, age information helpful in selecting the type of vaccine to administer, and insurance information if commercial insurance, Medicare, or

Medicaid are to be billed for the vaccine and immunization encounter. The individual responsible for consent documentation should have multiple copies of the forms, pens, and clipboards that can be disinfected. If electronic consent forms are to be used, this person can verify that the form has been completed and signed, if necessary. Paper copies of all forms should also be available. Individuals assigned to the job of consent documentation should have three responsibilities: 1) provide blank consent forms for vaccine recipients to complete while in their care, or review any completed consent forms they may have brought with them; 2) ask vaccine recipients to make available insurance information or money that will be collected at the finance station; and 3) verify the VIS is in the car and remind them to review after completing their consent documents.

The vaccination station is next in the process. It is here where the personnel performing the vaccination will be stationed along with the vaccine(s) and all vaccination supplies. Individuals working at this station will have critical responsibilities, so they must be able to work with as little distraction as possible. This group should consist of individuals who are competent to administer vaccines, assess the recipients, and lead emergency response activities, if necessary. Their three responsibilities include: 1) reviewing the patient consent documentation and clarifying responses that may indicate concerns regarding immunization or need to select specific vaccines (e.g., prior severe reaction to influenza vaccine, anaphylactic reaction to egg, adult over the age of 64); 2) selecting, administering, and documenting the correct vaccine for each recipient using best practice techniques; and 3) patient education post-vaccination. The VIS should guide patient education, so having the VIS readily available in the car enables the vaccinating individual to provide specific reference material and use it as a teaching adjunct.

The individual responsible for finance is the person who receives payment for the vaccine or gathers information necessary for billing to commercial insurance, Medicaid, or Medicare. If copies of insurance cards are to be obtained, there should be at least two small portable printers/scanners/copiers along with extra paper and toner cartridges. Several scanning applications can be used on mobile devices that may be a consideration. Since personal information is involved in transactions, the mobile device should be one that can protect that information. If cash is accepted, it is wise to price the vaccine charge amount, so it is easy to make change for larger bills. For example, avoid pricing vaccines at a cost that requires the return of multiple one-dollar bills. Targeting vaccine prices, so it is consistent with community pricing, is worth considering. If credit or debit cards are accepted, this person should have access to wireless transaction equipment and should be aware which, if any, credit cards are not accepted. Checks may present problems in the event any are returned for insufficient funds. Copies of receipts should indicate the clinic name, location, contact information, type of vaccine administered, lot number and expiration date, and cost. Receipts should have the signature of an individual who can respond to finance questions. The three responsibilities of the finance staff include: 1) obtaining insurance information or money for each dose of vaccine to be administered; 2) provide a receipt documenting the transaction; and 3) retrieval of the VIS from the car dashboard so they can be disinfected and reused. Payment for vaccination is either the easiest or the most challenging process for the drive-through. Devoting thought as to how transactions can be performed before the event (e.g., complete documentation online and pay online, or submit insurance information before the event) may save significant throughput and personnel time. If each person is to pay for their vaccine and be responsible for submitting to their insurer for reimbursement, they must be provided with a detailed receipt containing all information that will be requested of them. A detailed receipt should include CPT codes, vaccine names, administration codes, charges, the address of the clinic office, provider names, and identification codes such as their NPI number and tax ID of the office, along with the date of vaccine administration. To help preempt phone calls to the office, including the following items with the payment receipt is helpful, a list of Frequently Asked Questions (FAQs) outlining how to address issues with reimbursement, how to contact the office with questions, or how to report a post-vaccination concern or adverse event.

Patient education should be included throughout the entire process. Following vaccination, a designated educator should be responsible for three activities: 1) reinforcement of education provided by the vaccinator; 2) answering questions regarding the vaccination process; and 3) encouraging the vaccine recipient to pause for 10-15 minutes in a designated waiting area before exiting the property and provide information regarding "signals" they can use to call for assistance. Following vaccination, the recipient should receive specific information regarding their injection, including anticipated local reactions as well as systemic reactions that may occur. The VIS provides information to begin the conversation. Also, some patients may feel faint following an injection, often due to a vasovagal response. Although reports of adverse events identified during a drive-through vaccination event are infrequent, the individual responsible for patient education should be prepared for emergency response. The educator should also point vaccine recipients to a waiting area where they can remain for 10-15 minutes. Instructions such as "we would like for you to wait 15 minutes on-site [at the designated location]" may be useful. Although it is difficult to require this in a drive-through event, the educator can offer the option, and the logistics team can build in an exit route that maintains vaccine recipients on the property for minutes following vaccination. In large events, this waiting area may be a location for a first responder van or tent. For individual vehicles waiting in this area, they should be provided with information they can use to call for assistance if needed. These methods can include honking the horn or an arm visible outside the vehicle window.

Other personnel are needed for the drive-through in support roles, and one of these roles involves a vaccine monitor. This individual is responsible for the handling and management of the vaccine supplies. Their three responsibilities include 1) hourly temperature monitoring; 2) monitoring and maintaining adequate vaccine stock, and 3) moving vaccine from the vaccine refrigerator to the preparation area by the designated vaccinator(s). This is a critical role and should be handled by personnel attentive to detail. Hourly temperature monitoring must be performed and documented using forms that can be maintained and used as verification of the safe handling of the vaccine. This individual should monitor the flow of traffic through the drive-through and use that to monitor vaccine supply continuously. This includes monitoring types of vaccines if more than one is offered at the event (e.g., a different vaccine used for older adults) to ensure supply availability. Lastly, one person must be responsible for moving the vaccine from the refrigerator to the vaccination station. This helps ensure that vaccine is maintained in appropriate conditions until close to the time of vaccination. The timing of this movement is vital to protect the effectiveness of the vaccine. One approach that may be used is to provide an amount of vaccine that will be used within 30 minutes. This minimizes time outside the refrigerator and accidental mishandling in the event the vaccine is "forgotten". This individual should also monitor where the vaccine is located, so it is not in areas of excessive heat or cold or direct sunlight. As influenza vaccination events may occur during cold weather, the vaccine must never be exposed to freezing temperatures.

The supply monitor is responsible for ensuring that all supplies needed for the event are available and properly located. This job involves three responsibilities: 1) development of a supply list and daily event checklist to ensure supplies are available at the site; 2) placement of supplies at the various stations to ensure each has enough for that day's event activities; and 3) reconciliation of supplies available at the end of the day's event activities to ensure replacement and availability for the next event's needs. The supply monitor must work closely with the team leader and the finance individual for record keeping and documentation to ensure the replacement of supplies and ongoing availability.

Preventing infection in vaccine recipients and drive-through staff is the responsibility of the infection control monitor. This individual ensures that each station operates in a way that prevents transmission of infection to drive-through staff by monitoring the performance of hand hygiene, use of PPE, environmental disinfection, and safe injection practices. The three responsibilities of this role include: 1) assurance that supplies and equipment are available at each station and appropriately used; 2) active communication with personnel to identify "near miss" situations that have potential for harm and implementation of an immediate corrective plan and a report; and 3) ensuring any person experiencing exposure to blood or body fluids is immediately addressed and documented. Monitoring of practice is a continuous process and involves an open dialogue and reinforcement of the competency-based training provided for every person involved in the drive-through. More information regarding infection control is provided in Chapter 3.

Management of traffic will vary according to the size of the event and the venue itself. The individual responsible for traffic management will have these three responsibilities: 1) Supporting the pre-determined traffic flow patterns and working with the greeter to ensure uninterrupted traffic flow; 2) identifying bottlenecks in the tra c ow so corrective action can be taken, and 3) actively communicating with each station regarding tra c activity. This person will be mobile and likely move around the event site. They should stay in contact with the team leader and should have a way of communicating with each station. In a large event, communication equipment such as walkie-talkies is helpful.

Training

In terms of a multidisciplinary team, the team leader is the one designated to oversee the drive-through event. That role should be filled by a person planning to be on-site, ensuring all other team members are performing tasks as assigned. As we assemble our team that will help us implement a drive-through vaccine clinic, getting together to review a skills checklist, or perhaps sending participants a link to complete online training via the CDC website with information on which modules they are to complete is a good start. Discussing the "rights" of vaccination and the expectation as to each participant's role in the process is essential. Before the event, it should be confirmed that all personnel administering vaccines are certi ed in CPR and are familiar with the signs and symptoms of anaphylaxis. Everyone needs to know their role in an emergency, the location of epinephrine, and should be trained on epinephrine administration, this is discussed further in Chapter 7. The team leader must also ensure and document that the staff has the proper training for their role in vaccination. Safety procedures designed to prevent injury among personnel should be included in training for every position. Details such as not having personnel crossing between lanes when cars are moving and how to handle tents safely are essential points to include in training.

Some of the essential training points for personnel in each station are outlined below:

1)Greeter

- Clinic traffic plan
- VIS for each vaccine available for administration in the drive-through
- List of safety items necessary for the vehicle drivers including use of seat-belts, putting their vehicle in park at the vaccination station, ensuring children are in car seats and buckled in, preparing the arm for the injection by ensuring the area is exposed and without any tight sleeve or other restriction
- Techniques to address an anxious person
- Use of PPE and hand hygiene performance

2)Consent and documentation

- Addressing questions vaccine recipients may have as they complete the consent or data collection form
- Handling questions when they are unsure of the correct answer(s)
- Guiding individuals in the vehicle regarding safe ways to complete documentation forms while also moving forward in the queue
- Approaches to obtaining additional supplies (e.g., copies of consent forms, pens, clipboards)
- Use of PPE and hand hygiene performance

3)Vaccinator

- Knowledge of all vaccines to be provided in the drive-through event including information provided on the VIS
- Handling of the vaccine including multi-dose vials (MDV) and prefilled syringes
- Use of personal protective equipment and hand hygiene performance
- Principles of asepsis and ensuring a clear separation of clean items from dirty items
- Environmental infection control
- Infection control including wiping of MDV septum before withdrawing any dose of vaccine
- Injection landmarks
- Skin disinfection
- Injection site selection, correct syringe and needle size, and injection techniques
- Administration of intranasal vaccine, if offered in the drive-through
- Post-vaccination site care
- Patient education including information regarding a follow-up dose for children under the age of nine if this is their first influenza vaccination

- Documentation of vaccine brand, expiration date, lot number, injection site location
- Emergency response

4)Finance

- Working knowledge regarding insurance billing and the documentation necessary for payment submission to commercial insurers, Medicaid and Medicare
- Ability to respond to frequently asked questions vaccine recipients may have concerning insurance
- Equipment used at the drive-through for credit card payments
- Monitoring process for the security of any cash, check or credit card payments
- Information security practices to protect the personal and health information of all vaccine recipients
- Use of personal protective equipment and hand hygiene performance

5)Patient educator

- Knowledge regarding all vaccines to be administered in the drive-through event and anticipated vaccine reactions
- Managing an anxious vaccine recipient
- Emergency response
- Use of personal protective equipment and hand hygiene performance

6)Vaccine monitor

- Knowledge regarding all vaccines to be administered in the drive-through event and anticipated vaccine reactions
- Awareness of all vaccine expiration dates and a list of all vaccines including supply level
- Temperature requirements for all vaccine and the associate documentation information and forms
- Vaccine refrigerator operation
- Data logger temperature monitor operation
- Use of personal protective equipment and hand hygiene performance

7)Supply monitor

- Awareness of all supplies to be used in the drive-through event
- Supply levels and any special care required for any supply (e.g., maintaining a closed top in any environmental pop-up wipe, avoiding moisture contact with sterile supplies)
- Pre-determined transport process to move supplies from a designated holding area to the station at which supplies will be used

- Use of PPE and hand hygiene performance

8) Infection control monitor

- Knowledge regarding basic infection control practice
- Knowledge of safe injection practice
- Process for identifying practice deviation and initiating immediate correction
- Environmental infection control
- Use of personal protective equipment and hand hygiene performance

9) Traffic management

- Awareness of the traffic pattern when on-site at the venue
- Contact information in the event traffic congestion occurs, and there is a recognized impact on local traffic on-site of the venue
- Managing the anxious vaccine recipient
- General safety practices introduced and reinforced by the greeter
- Ability to identify impending safety issues and determine a safe response
- Use of personal protective equipment and hand hygiene performance

We cannot underestimate the need for "runners" or ancillary staff to be able to handle things as they come up. It is crucial to make sure that people assigned have the ability to carry out these roles when asked to perform them. They need to understand what they're expected to do, where to find things, and that they are empowered to handle that. It may be that they assist with the critical task of handling vaccines if they have been trained to do so, field patient questions, traffic control, assisting with the financial component, and helping with supplies. As mentioned, ensuring that vaccine recipients are waiting approximately 15 minutes following vaccination helps make sure everyone is doing well while waiting for departure.

Working in a small clinic with limited personnel and having the goal to implement something on a larger scale leaves many gaps to fill. Partnerships may be the key to successful implementation. Personnel that work in emergency management have a responsibility to test that role regularly to see how well it works. This is an ideal situation to put that into practice so that when emergencies do occur, they have had an opportunity to practice the skill set of crowd or incident control, traffic control, and the like. School systems with school nurses and schools of nursing may also be other avenues to pursue assistance with such an event. To enlist the support of others in your endeavor, you may find that staff come with a broad range of experience. Still, it is essential to convey that there is a competency-based training program you must implement and document, and there may be policies and procedures in place specific to your organization that must be adhered to. It is crucial in competency-based training, especially for vaccine preparation and administration, that we train to implement. The goal must be to provide a safe environment and prevent vaccine administration errors.

An excellent resource that can be used to assess and document competence is the "Skills Checklist for Vaccine Administration" by the Immunization Action Coalition. This document is included in the tools and resource section of this chapter. If you are recruiting assistance from individuals outside your organization with healthcare experience, but unsure about their baseline vaccination experience, this is an excellent tool to be able to begin an assessment. It applies more to a clinical setting but can certainly be adapted for a drive-through use. There are many great practical tools and visual resources offered by this organization, including frequently asked questions about a variety of vaccines that can be accessed on their website.

The rights of medication or vaccine administration have evolved and have no doubt grown longer, depending on when a person started their career in nursing. It is essential to know how you plan to tailor staff training utilizing this important tool. <u>Right Patient:</u> Two identifiers minimum. Unfortunately, those of us in healthcare could list untold stories of things that can go wrong by not identifying the correct patient and how easily that can happen. <u>Right Time:</u> f a four-year-old presents to a drive-through flu clinic and the parent requests the live intranasal flu vaccine, but we have failed to screen this patient, and they received the second MMR two weeks ago, the live intranasal vaccine is considered an invalid dose. The correct minimum interval comes into play when two live viruses are administered less than 28 days apart. Also, if it is a child's first flu season, they are recommended to receive a second dose of influenza vaccine a minimum of four weeks after the first. Understanding the spacing and timing of vaccines is critical to getting it right the first time and preventing a vaccine administration error.

When the plan is to recruit a small cadre of well-trained volunteers to assist with a larger immunization clinic, you will review with this group how to screen patients to give the right vaccine. In terms of screening, a patient reporting a history of Guillain-Barre Syndrome, within six weeks following an influenza vaccine, should be deferred on vaccinating in this type of setting at this time until it is known or confirmed through follow-up with a provider familiar with the patient's history, as to whether they are truly unable to receive the vaccine. Having a cold or the sniffles would not be a cause to miss an opportunity to vaccinate. If a patient states they have rare anaphylaxis to eggs, there is an influenza product available for that patient. However, most patients with an "egg allergy" can receive influenza vaccines without concern. Pregnancy will preclude one from receiving the live intranasal vaccine. If there is a question as to whether a patient could be pregnant, provide the inactivated vaccine via intramuscular injection. When the strategy is to provide patients with a precision immunization approach, consider that over the age of 65, due to immunosenescence, we may offer patients a high dose or adjuvanted vaccine. Keep in mind that the CDC does not have a preferential stance on types of vaccines. An individual who is immunocompromised by disease or medication and will not respond to a standard influenza vaccine with the same immune response as the general population should also be considered for a high dose or adjuvanted influenza vaccine.

Depending on what brand of influenza vaccine, the right dosage may vary for age group six through 35 months. The correct dosage for one brand is 0.25 mL, while another is 0.5 mL. Double-check this before the vaccination event and ensure safeguards are in place to prevent incorrect dose administration. You may decide it is easier to have only one brand of standard influenza vaccine that is suitable for ages six months and older. The intranasal flu vaccine is 0.1 mL in each nostril for a total of 0.2 mL dosage. The divider clip is what is used to determine the forced stopping point for the first push of the plunger. Removing the clip will allow the deployment of the remaining half dose by continuing with a second spray into the next nostril.

Once again, the Immunization Action Coalition has an excellent reference table for needle size based on age, sex, and weight. This right needle, route, and technique information is also included in the tools and resource section of this chapter. In a drive-through scenario where children are receiving vaccinations, a vaccinator must quickly assess in a toddler between the ages of one and three years, the amount of muscle mass and ease of exposing an area, as to whether the anterolateral thigh or deltoid muscle of the arm is the preferred site. Information on route, technique, and injection site will be reviewed in more extensive detail in subsequent chapters.

Federal law outlines the right documentation requirement that must be included in a person's record when administering a vaccine. This consists of the brand name of the vaccine, the manufacturer, lot number, VIS edition, date VIS given, date vaccine administered, name and title of person administering, and where administered. The name, clinic address, and telephone number can be preprinted on the information given to the patient. In addition to the provider's electronic health record, the Immunization Information System (IIS will be the place that this information can be accessed by the patient and other providers in perpetuity. The IIS will be discussed in extensive detail in another chapter. When patients or providers are unable to access documentation of a vaccine record, this can lead to unnecessary vaccines, incorrect spacing, or missed opportunities to complete needed vaccinations.

The role an individual will be assigned for the vaccination clinic will drive recommendations for the use of PPE, especially when addressing vaccination and COVID-19. The CDC's Advisory Committee on Immunization Practices (ACIP) will generally indicate that when administering immunizations, it is not necessary to wear gloves. Loss of manual dexterity has the potential to increase the risk of needle stick injuries. However, if a vaccinator has open sores, cracks, or cuts in the skin, gloves should be worn. When administering the intranasal influenza vaccine, staff may not have worn gloves in previous years. However, during this time of COVID-19 and the contact with a patient's face and possibly nasal secretions, gloves should be donned for this type of administration. Upon completion of vaccination, gloves should be removed, and hand hygiene performed.

Due to having close contact with a multitude of patients, while administering immunizations in a drive-through setting, gowns, surgical masks or respirators, and face shields may be necessary as part of the COVID-19 response, which was never considered necessary previously. Guidance on the use of PPE may vary based upon the positivity rate or the number of positive cases in a particular location. Public health recommendations should be sought when planning for the drive-through event while in its earliest stages.

In a large-scale drive-through setting, where the need to move vehicles quickly through the queue will be a necessity; it may not be feasible to have clients turn the car engine off completely. Forced air such as A/C or heat should be shut down so as not to create a positive pressure environment with air from the car cabin being forcefully directed at the vaccinator. Vaccinating children or administering the intranasal influenza vaccine can most certainly be an aerosol-generating procedure! Both of these examples demonstrate the need to strongly consider the wearing of face shields, in addition to masks, by all involved in the vaccination process.

When reviewing additional skills, focus with staff, make sure to review the use of aseptic technique, especially when using multi-dose vials, which must be disinfected before each entry. Monitoring vaccine temperature will be covered in extensive detail in Chapter 5. Staff must understand the importance of this role if assigned. Ensure that individuals are receiving good vaccines by maintaining viable temperatures. Proper hand hygiene between each person is essential. Plenty of hand sanitizers should be available (at least 60% ethyl or isopropyl alcohol), and gloves (if worn) must be changed in between each person vaccinated.

Protecting health information may include keeping forms secure in totes, upside down with paperweights, avoiding any sort of cumulative sign-in forms, and reiterating for staff that although healthcare is being provided in an alternate setting, privacy and protecting health information (PHI) rules still apply.

CHAPTER 3

DRIVE-THROUGH VACCINATION: INFECTION CONTROL AND SAFE INJECTION PRACTICES

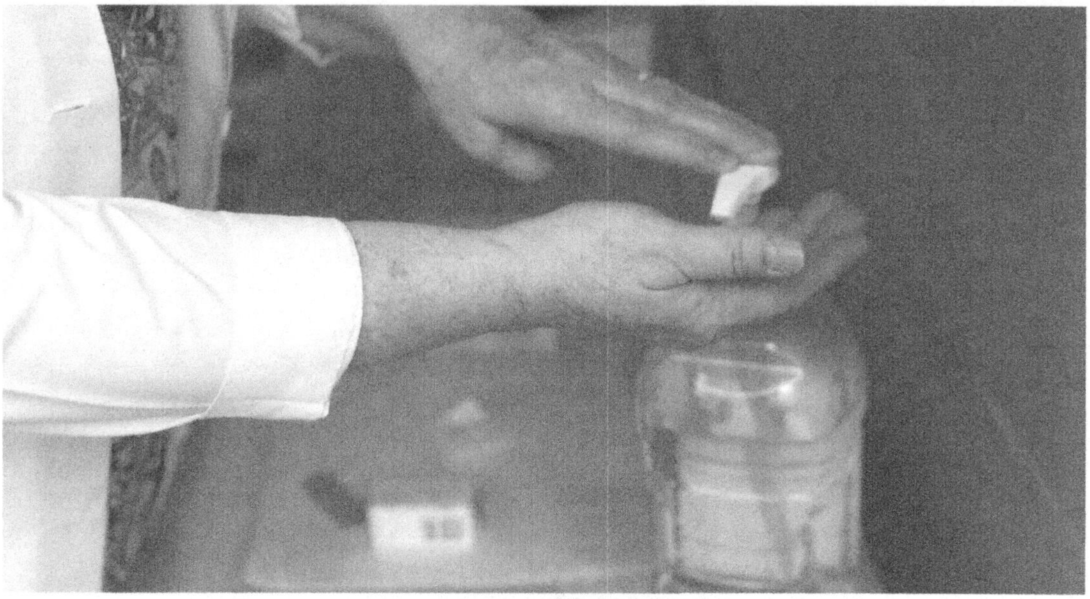

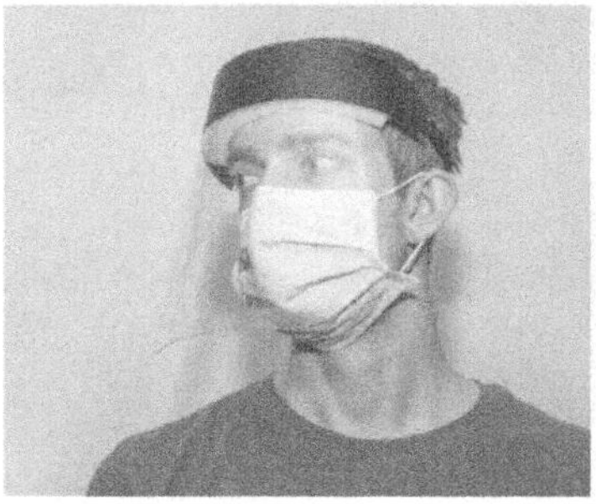

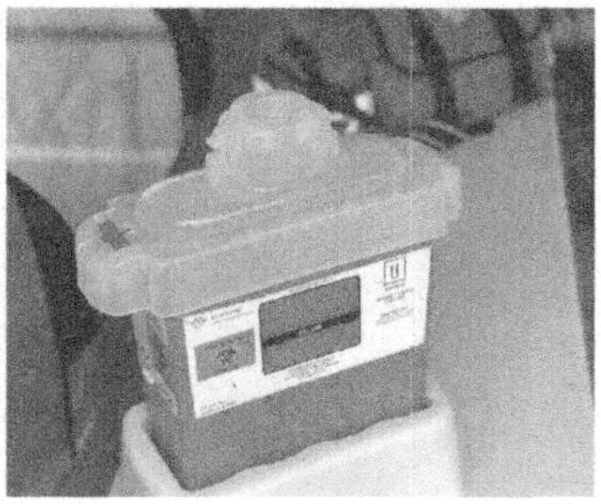

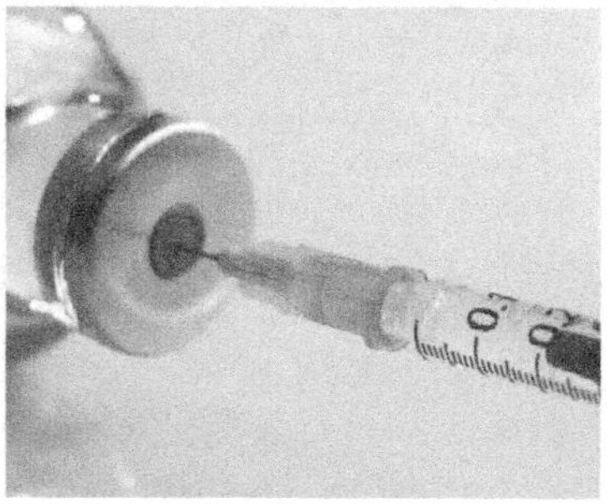

Hudson Garrett PhD MPH MBA FNP-BC, Ruth Carrico PhD DNP FNP-C

Preventing infection among personnel planning and implementing the drive-through vaccination event as well as preventing infection among vaccine recipients are critical program elements. Addressing infection control during the time of COVID-19 has magnified this importance. It has also demonstrated the need to consider additional use of personal protective equipment as part of vaccination that has not previously been considered a part of routine immunization. To address these issues, the review of infection control for drive-through vaccination will include: 1) basics of infection prevention and control and exposure prevention and management relevant in a drive-through vaccination event, and 2) safe injection practices for vaccines administered in a drive-through event. Two essential resources for this chapter include the CDC's Core Infection Prevention and Control practices relevant for care provided in all settings and the CDC's ACIP General Best Practice Guidelines for Immunization.

Infection Prevention and Control

When planning and implementing a drive-through vaccination clinic, basic infection control practices that must be addressed in training and competence verification include the following:

- Hand hygiene
- Environmental cleaning and disinfection
- Aseptic technique
- Proper use of Personal Protective Equipment (PPE)
- Mitigation of sharps injuries and exposure to blood or body fluids

Hand hygiene

Access to sinks may be limited at the station where vaccinations will occur during a drive-through. Alcohol-based hand rub should be immediately available at every station. Larger containers that prevent the need for the vaccinators to bend and stoop to access may help minimize complaints of sore back muscles due to that repetitive movement. Bottled water should also be available in the event exposure to blood or body fluid occurs, and a wash is needed to immediately remove that fluid and cleanse the exposed area(s). Personnel must have knowledge of and demonstrate competence in hand hygiene performance, including when to perform, how to perform, and how often to perform. Gloves are not generally worn during vaccination events, but COVID-19 may change that approach for some clinics. If gloves are worn, they should be changed after every patient, and hand hygiene performed after removal.

Environmental cleaning and disinfection

Environmental surfaces such as tabletops and shared items can serve as reservoirs for pathogens and lead to potential contamination and subsequent transmission. Any tables or counters that are used to store supplies for the drive-through should be cleaned and disinfected at setup and the end of the event day. If visible soil is present or if there are questions about contamination, the surface should be disinfected more frequently. An approach to environmental cleaning and disinfection helps ensure surfaces are maintained throughout the event to prevent contamination of supplies or exposure to personnel. All disinfectants used in the US must be regulated and registered by the US Environmental Protection Agency (EPA). A broad-spectrum, hospital-grade disinfectant should be used to clean and disinfect all environmental surfaces and equipment (e.g., outside of the vaccine refrigerator before packing and after transport). Care must also be taken to follow the overall contact time for the selected disinfectant and allow the surface to remain wet for the manufacturer's recommended contact time. Complete instructions for disinfectants may be obtained from the product's label and also on the EPA website in the form of the EPA Master Label. When using pop-up disinfectant wipes, the contact time is often clearly displayed on the outside of the container. Contact times may range from 1-10 minutes, so carefully read the product label to know how to use the wipes, so they are effective. Concerning COVID-19, the EPA maintains a List N that has products deemed as effective against this virus. However, it is crucial to recognize that this virus is easily inactivated by the hospital-grade disinfectants routinely used in most healthcare facilities. List N germicides can be viewed by going to the EPA website.

Aseptic technique

The principles of asepsis focus on the constant and consistent separation of clean from dirty. This means that clean equipment is separated from items that have been used. In a drive-through vaccination event, unused injection equipment and supplies, vaccines, unused PPE, and hand hygiene products should be completely separated from the regular trash, regulated waste, and sharps containers. Separate areas for vaccination preparation should be prepared, regularly disinfected, and monitored to ensure safety for the vaccine recipient. The flow of activity should follow the "clean to dirty" approach. This means that the clean area where sterile and clean supplies are handled should be together and located, so they are readily available to the vaccinator. Once vaccination has occurred, the "dirty" areas where trash is placed and sharps containers are located should be away from the clean area and placed, so personnel does not have to cross the "dirty" area to access the "clean" area. Using simulation and the use of graphic drawings can help outline the flow of the items and activities, so all personnel understands the aseptic approach.

Personal Protective Equipment (PPE)

Before COVID-19, rarely was PPE used as part of vaccination regardless of whether it occurred in a routine office or pharmacy clinic or via a drive-through approach. The OSHA guidance for PPE use involved whether contact with blood or body fluid could be reasonably anticipated. CDC guidance provided through the standard precautions recommendations mirrored the OSHA approach. If you could reasonably expect contact with blood or body fluid, you selected PPE based upon that interaction. The use of gloves as part of vaccination has not been a CDC recommendation and aligned with reasonable anticipation as contact with blood should be a rare event when using competent practice. When administering an intramuscular injection, if the muscle is relaxed and there are no restricting clothing providing that "tourniquet effect," bleeding at the injection site following removal of the needle should be the exception rather than the rule. Having a readily available 2x2 to apply over the injection site and a Band-Aid to cover the site following removal of the 2x2 is a way to add to the unlikely event blood is present following the injection.

COVID-19 has caused us to consider how to safely provide vaccination at a time when recipients may be ill, or if either the recipient or the healthcare worker is asymptomatic or per-symptomatic carriers of the virus. This has resulted in the need to reconsider PPE use as part of routine practice during a drive-through vaccination event. In these situations, PPE should be worn to prevent contact with respiratory droplets that can be projected from a vaccine recipient to the healthcare worker AS WELL AS from the healthcare worker to the vaccine recipient or others in their vehicle. Healthcare worker to healthcare worker transmission must also be considered. Therefore, recognizing the close contact that may occur among individuals in a vaccination drive-through and recognizing PPE may be worn for prolonged periods, a safe approach would involve the use of masks and face shields by drive-through personnel. An N95 respirator could be worn, but it is essential to recognize that respirators may be more difficult for the healthcare worker to tolerate for prolonged periods and use for extended periods may result in more face touching and other transmission-prone activities. Gloves could be beneficial if the healthcare worker is administering the intranasal vaccine due to the close proximity of their hands to the nose and mouth of the vaccine recipient. It can be reasonably anticipated that hands, in that circumstance, are at risk for contamination with respiratory droplets. Gloves could be worn, and hand hygiene performed following their immediate removal once vaccination is complete for that individual recipient to minimize contamination. The need for gowns is likely to be unnecessary but is an acceptable PPE addition if personnel so choose. If worn, gowns should be removed at predetermined intervals (e.g., anytime the personnel leaves the vaccination area for a break, at the end of a shift, anytime the gown is visibly soiled or there is concern about contamination) and disposed of in regular trash receptacles. Discussion with local public health will help determine if more widespread PPE is needed or recommended. Ultimately, there must be a risk-benefit discussion and competency-based training to ensure the workers can select, put on, wear, remove, and dispose of PPE safely. Hand hygiene must always follow PPE removal.

Mitigation of sharps injuries and exposure

Engineering controls must be in place to minimize the opportunity for occupational exposure involving blood or body fluids. Safety needles, sharps containers that are not overfilled, and availability of PPE to provide barrier precaution are examples of prevention and mitigation strategies. Providing vaccination with the recipient in the vehicle is also a mitigation strategy as the recipient can be asked to put on their mask or face covering and turn their head away from the drive-through personnel. Vehicle environmental adjustments, including opening windows and turning off the heat/AC fan, minimizes the blowing of air from inside the vehicle into the face of the drive-through personnel. The use of PPE also helps mitigate exposure risk. If, however, any personnel report an exposure event, there must be a predetermined approach for immediate evaluation and intervention by a healthcare provider specializing in exposure events. An occupational health nurse, infection preventionist, or infectious diseases nurse practitioner or physician are several examples.

Safe Injection Practice

Safe Injection practices are a crucial element in maintaining the safety of all vaccines and those who receive them and those who administer them. Safe injection practices relevant to vaccine administration during a drive-through event include the following:

- Hand hygiene
- Withdrawing vaccine from a multi-dose vial (MDV)
- Single-use of all injection components including syringe and needle
- Connecting sterile needles to sterile syringes
- Conditions under which vaccines are stored and transported
- Injection technique
- Handling and disposal of used injection items

Hand hygiene

Hands should be cleansed prior to gathering or touching any items involved in the injection. Hand washing is an ideal activity but may not be consistently possible in a drive-through vaccination event. Therefore, alcohol-based hand rubs should be immediately available and placed in the area where vaccine and vaccination supplies are handled.

Withdrawing vaccine from a multi-dose vial (MDV)

A new sterile needle and syringe must be used for every dose of vaccine withdrawn from any vial. If an MDV of vaccine is used, it is essential to disinfect the top of the vial (diaphragm) with an alcohol swab. A practice of using a resealable bag with cotton balls soaked in alcohol is unacceptable. Hands going in and out of the bag results in contamination, and that level of contamination may exceed the disinfecting capabilities of the alcohol. Only sterile alcohol swabs should be used and, once used, discarded. Friction should be used for approximately 10 seconds to disinfect the diaphragm using a single sterile alcohol swab. Then, a sterile syringe and sterile needle can be inserted through the diaphragm and a single dose of vaccine withdrawn. For each subsequent dose of vaccine withdrawn from the vial, the diaphragm is again scrubbed with a new sterile alcohol swab, and a new sterile syringe and sterile needle are used to draw the next dose. Vials will contain a small amount of overfill designed to accommodate dead space volumes of various syringe types and needles. The pooling of any overfill amount of leftover vaccine from one vial is never to be mixed with the vaccine in another vial to achieve a complete dose volume. Excess vaccine that is less than a full dose should be discarded.

Single-use of all injection components including syringe and needle

Sterile single-use needles and syringes must be used for every dose of vaccine. Reuse of any item is unacceptable and represents possible harm. Needle technology is designed to retain its "sharpness", so there is no need to change needles before injection even though the sterile needle has been used to pierce the MDV diaphragm. Changing needles provides an opportunity for contamination and should be avoided. Smaller gauge needles take longer to withdraw vaccines simply due to physics, but this does not indicate the need to change needles.

Connecting sterile needles to sterile syringes

When using a sterile prefilled syringe, only a new sterile needle should be attached in preparation for injection. Prefilled syringes, like single-dose vials, do not contain preservatives. The goal of the preservative is to prevent microbial growth in the vaccine. Prefilled syringes and single-dose vials are packaged under sterile conditions at the pharmaceutical company. Once a needle is connected to the prefilled syringe, that results in the "activation" of the syringe. The sterile conditions in place at the time of packaging have been altered, and the vaccine should, therefore, be administered as soon as possible. It is never acceptable to put needles on multiple prefilled syringes in preparation for administration. This enables contamination opportunities and the potential for harm.

Conditions under which vaccines are stored and transported

Vaccines should be stored and transported in their original containers. Packaging protects the vials and syringes from contact resulting in cracking of vials or prefilled syringe hubs. The original packaging also enables a controlled temperature of the vaccine and protection from direct contact with transport-approved cold or frozen packs. If "activated" syringes are transported, there are opportunities for contamination during transport, especially if the syringes contact moisture. This is why it is never acceptable to transport vaccines (or other sterile medication or items) in coolers with ice as the melting ice facilitates microbial contamination of the syringe and its needle and contents, this is discussed in detail in Chapter 5.

Injection technique

Sterile needles should be unsheathed immediately before injection. Never walk around with an exposed needle. Not only can this result in unrecognized contamination, but it may also serve to increase anxiety among the vaccine recipients. Care must be taken to ensure that the needle does not contact the hands of the healthcare worker or any other item before injection if a sterile needle is applied to the hub of a prefilled syringe. Care must be taken to ensure that the fingertips of the one applying the sterile needle avoid contact with the sterile hub area of the syringe. This constitutes the traditional "no-touch zone". If such contact occurs, the needle and the vaccine must be discarded.

Handling and disposal of used injection items

Once the injection has occurred, the safety device of the needle must be activated immediately after removing the needle from the recipient. This immediate action protects the vaccinator from accidental needle stick. The needle and syringe must be placed directly into a sharps container. In a drive-through vaccination event, it is helpful if items are placed, so the need to bend and stop is minimized. Tall sharps containers, or those in a stabilizing stand placed on a table, are preferable. Sharps containers should be closed and replaced once they reach the indicator line on the container. This prevents overfilling and the potential for inadvertent contact with over ow injection items.

Even when all infection prevention and control and safe injection practices are closely followed, there is always a potential risk for an unexpected adverse event. This may occur when conducting a drive-through vaccination event or when performing vaccination in a traditional office or pharmacy setting. A proactive response plan should incorporate current recommendations from the Centers for Disease Control and Prevention (CDC), including:

- Designating a specific individual to provide ongoing oversight for infection control
- Developing written infection control policies and procedures
- Providing role-specific and competency-based training for all personnel involved in the event
- Periodic observations of infection control practices and providing immediate feedback to personnel as a corrective measure

In the event, there is an infection control or safe injection practice breach, and it is crucial to have a notification plan in place. The CDC has created an excellent resource entitled the Patient Notification Toolkit. This serves as a comprehensive guide to best practices used to communicate adverse events to patients, the public, and the media. The team leader should consider designating a team member to act as the media liaison.

The key to achieving excellence in infection prevention and control and safe injection practice is to maintain constant vigilance for breaches in practice and continuously assess clinical practices. Those served by drive-through vaccination clinics have the same expectation of safe clinical care as they would have when seeking care in their primary care office. Infection control is everyone's responsibility, and it is through that shared accountability that the safety of all can be assured and maintained.

CHAPTER 4

DRIVE-THROUGH VACCINATION: VACCINE AND INVENTORY MANAGEMENT

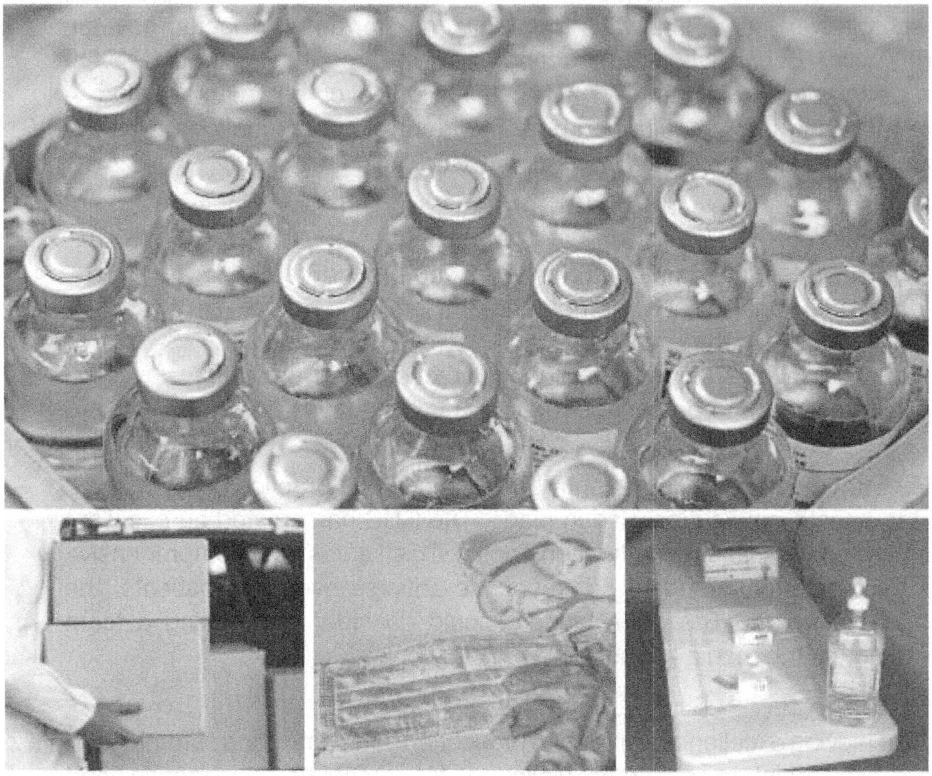

Luanne Didelot MHA MSN, Ruth Carrico PhD DNP FNP-C

Determining vaccine types and amounts during a drive-through event can be a bit tricky when pivoting to an entirely different vaccination process and format. If a particular event, such as a drive-through, is "open-ended" to any degree as to the number that may choose to participate, or if a clinic is trying to determine the amount of vaccine to order for the upcoming flu season without a reasonable estimate as to the expected uptake, a few strategies come to mind. Determining the amounts administered during the previous year's influenza season would be a good baseline and adjust accordingly. Inquiring from your vaccine representative as to the return policy for unused vaccines or setting up a system to query the patient population should help get a handle on expected numbers. Partnering with another clinic to "borrow" or "transfer" vaccine may be an alternative.

Consider the general age of your population served. Will a pediatric population be more inclined toward FluMist®? Will you expect to see a larger older adult or retired population, and does that mean you need to have several different types of influenza vaccine available. If you are able to administer in a drive-through with a perceived "safer" environment than traditional settings, will that result in more older adults with mobility issues as well as families with multiple children and concerns about bringing them as a group into a traditional office setting? These types of considerations are important to discuss with your planning team as you determine types of vaccines and amounts.

Referencing a list of vaccine products may help determine the number of supplies needed. Prefilled syringes will require only the needle, while Multi-Dose Vials (MDV) will, of course, require the use of a needle and syringe. Anticipating the number of other supplies needed will be based on vaccines administered, including Band-Aids, 2x2's, and alcohol prep pads for each vaccination and enough extra to wipe the septum of the MDV with every entry. Prefilled syringes for large vaccination clinics are the obvious choice due to ease of use. However, the increased cost may be a consideration.

Anticipating the different types and sizes of needles will be based upon the population expected to participate. It is easier and acceptable to bring more ancillary supplies than anticipated, so there are no issues. Transporting a temperature-sensitive vaccine will be a more judicious process. Reviewing your list of syringe types and needle sizes, which vary based on age, weight, and sex, will need to be taken into consideration when determining a "packing list." The emergency kit and protocol will be required for all off-site vaccination clinics. The contents must be reviewed to ensure the appropriate medications are included, and expiration dates have been reviewed. An example of a supply list is included in the tools and resource section of this chapter.

The immunization protocol for the vaccines to be administered, standing orders (if applicable), screening tools, vaccine information statements (VIS) for each vaccine to be administered, extra forms, and the patient immunization record provided to the patient should be included in items taken to the clinic. Temperature logs for each vaccine bag or refrigerator/freezer will be needed to document the vaccine temperature hourly while at off-site clinics.

Tissues are always good to have that on hand, especially if you're administering the live attenuated influenza vaccine (LAIV) FluMist, and disinfecting wipes for cleaning tables. Fast-acting carbohydrates (15 grams) may be helpful for people with low blood sugar and others who complain of feeling lightheaded or shaky. Regular (not diet) soda can go along way for someone weak in the knees! In most instances, those situations are mitigated by the fact that people are seated, in a comfortable environment, in their vehicle. Treats, stickers, or dog treats are also a welcome thing!

Managing inventory is aided by a checklist that includes the items and can also include the amount of stock you plan for the drive-through event. This can also serve as a base document for financial planning, documenting, and reconciliation. The utilization of prefilled syringes is a helpful strategy in making the process of drawing up and administering vaccines quicker and less error-prone. However, there will be a slight difference in cost, with the MDV often being cheaper. Discussing ahead of time with individuals in your clinic that oversee vaccine ordering and those that are responsible for the financial function and providing an understanding of how the process of administration works and the scenarios in which is product may be best utilized is vital. There may be specific situations in which your clinic may use both types of products, depending on which situation is more appropriate. With any vaccination event, it will be critical to think about having protocols in place to reduce opportunities for patient harm. If there is not a controlled and clean environment to be able to draw up a vaccine out of the multi-dose vial, you might consider, from a patient safety perspective, the decision to use only prefilled syringes in that setting.

Another advantage of preflled syringe is that it generally has a removable label.

This label can be peeled off he barrel of the syringe and used to quickly and accurately document lot number, type of vaccine, and other required information in a very efficient way. This is not provided for vaccine drawn from an MDV, so preprinted labels could be useful. Color-coding is a helpful way of keeping track of different types of vaccines and preventing error.

Re-dose needs should always be considered when ordering the vaccine. What will the process be for children under the age of nine who have not had two doses of influenza vaccine previously and are required to have a second dose? How will that be handled, and by whom?

The graphic representing the types of vaccine errors included in the tools and resource section of this chapter illustrates that it is critically important when having different types and brands of the vaccine in your inventory, that staff retrained to screen for age/indications/contraindications/allergies, proper spacing of doses, dosages, and administration routes.

Packing Checklist: Off-Site Vaccination Clinic

- Approved portable plug-in refrigerator and/or freezer OR vaccine transport bag
- Digital Data Logger and Buffered Probe
- Off-site temperature logs (on per qualified container or pack-out)
- Vaccine
- 1mL syringes, if using Multi-Dose Vials (MDV)
- Needles: Pediatric and Adult (5/8", 1" and 1 ½")
- Alcohol pads
- 2x2s
- Band-Aids
- Emergency kit and printed protocol
- Immunization protocol for the vaccine(s) to be administered
- Vaccine Information Statements for all vaccines to be administered
- Screening forms
- Extra consent forms / pens / clipboards
- Patient immunization record or card to provide vaccine information
- Tissue box
- Disinfecting wipes
- Table covers (paper or paper with uid-resistant backing)
- Hand sanitizer (60% ethyl or isopropyl alcohol)
- Sharps containers
- Medical waste bags/ trash bags
- PPE as indicated (synthetic exam gloves, masks, face shield, gowns)
- Fast-acting carbohydrate (regular soda [not diet], glucose tablets, Smarties, cake gel)
- Treats / Stickers / Doggie Treats!
- Prepared statement of the address location and telephone number of the event location in the cellphone of all team members in case EMS needs to be activated

CHAPTER 5

DRIVE-THROUGH VACCINATION: VACCINE STORAGE, TRANSPORT AND TEMPERATURE MONITORING

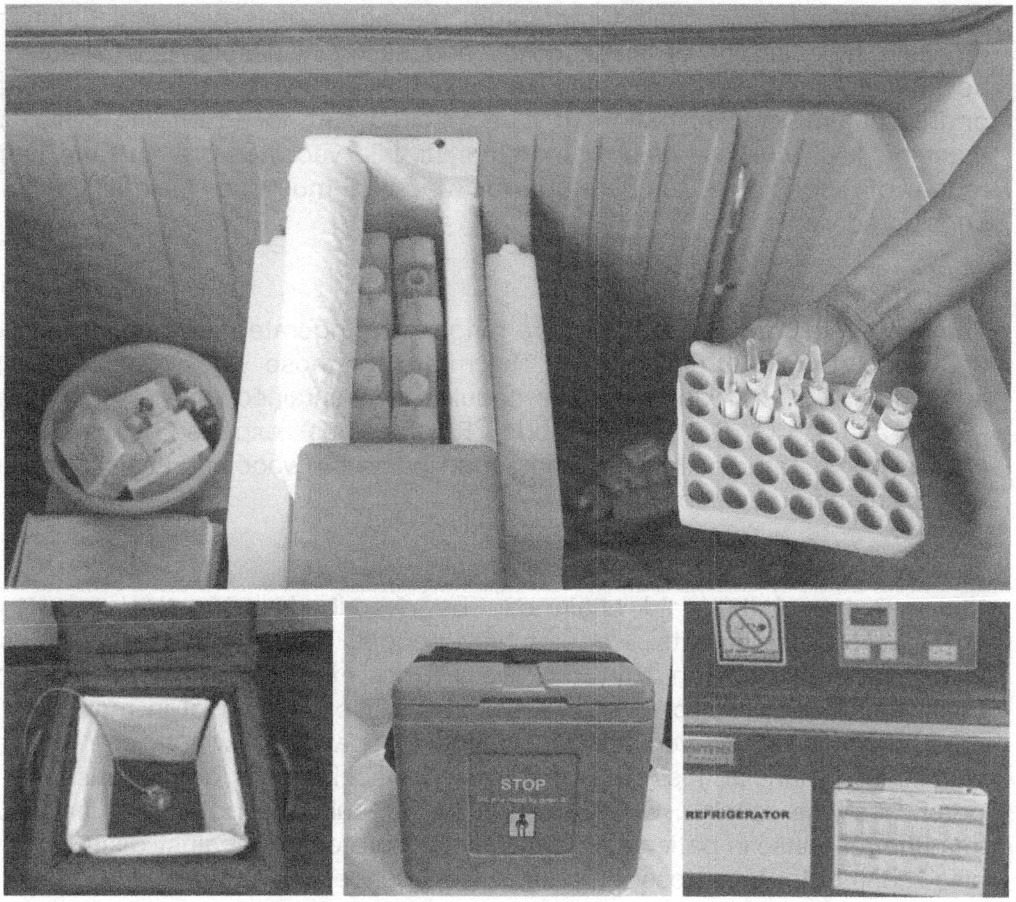

Luanne Didelot MHA MSN, Ruth Carrico PhD DNP FNP-C

Strategies for managing the cold chain become more complex and critical when vaccinating in a mobile setting. Vaccine temperature monitoring and the associated documentation can prevent "excursions", which is a very fancy way of saying the vaccine became either too hot or too cold. It was outside the acceptable temperature range for fragile vaccines. The "Cold Chain Flowchart" is taken from the CDC Storage and Handling Toolkit. The cold chain is defined as the temperature management of vaccines from the time they leave the production, all the way up until the dose is administered to the patient. Vaccine cold chain temperature management is a critical function to maintain the viability of these costly and essential assets. It is affected by how we store and handle the vaccine, including removing from the refrigerator or freezer until administration. If it is "packed-out" to an off-site clinic, staff must be keenly aware of how extremely fragile vaccines are and the narrow range of acceptable temperature in which it must be maintained to be considered viable.

The acceptable vaccine temperature range for refrigerated vaccines is between 2°C and 8°C OR 36°F and 46°F. The motto for those who manage vaccines is "strive for 5"! Frozen vaccines should be maintained at a temperature of -50°C and -15°C OR -58°F and 5°F. Vaccines exposed to colder or warmer temperatures than recommended place the vaccines at risk, and they may be rendered ineffective.

Management of the cold chain can be described within the con nes of three essential elements: equipment, people, systems and processes. If there is a breakdown in any area, we will not experience a good, tight cold chain that is required for best practice vaccination. Our goal in managing the cold chain is to prevent re-vaccination of patients, which can cause a significant financial loss due to wasted vaccines, a compromise in the potency of the vaccine, which may, in turn, result in a potentially inadequate immune response in patients, and insufficient protection against disease. It can also contribute to a loss of patient confidence in vaccines and providers, which is counterproductive to the mission of public health.

"People" are the individuals involved in the handling process from manufacturing, to distribution, to clinic employees that accept the shipments and monitor the vaccine refrigerators/freezers, up to the healthcare personnel administering the vaccine. This seems to be one of the most variable components of the process, which should be addressed with training and experience. A clinic that maintains a small cadre of people, very well trained in vaccination, is the ultimate scenario as opposed to expecting everyone to have some knowledge or "a hand in the process". From the minute a shipment arrives in a clinic, staff must appreciate how controlled the process of vaccine management must be.

Equipment refers to items including vaccine refrigerators, freezers, pack-out containers, data loggers, and shipping containers. An excellent training tool is the CDC Module 10: Storage and Handling. This module can be accessed through the public health learning management system, TRAIN. Providers who are enrolled, and those that handle Vaccine for Children (VFC), are required to complete this online training module annually and maintain documentation of training.

When we highlight the enormous benefit of training, it is also important to remember that providers need to empower those in their clinic to identify problems and be able to respond to them. There is a distinct difference between recognizing a problem and responding to what has been identified. It does not benefit an office or the patient to recognize a problem and not implement corrective action. It is imperative that everyone involved in any part of the immunization process strive for the same goal, and that is making sure our actions do not result in patient harm. If we immunize with a vaccine that has not been appropriately cared for, the vaccine itself may not hurt them, but the whole notion that we failed to protect them when we had the opportunity, that is, the patient harm. So every person, as part of the process, should be looking to identify an error or error-prone system or process. There should then be a clear directive that once a problem has been identified, we need to ensure we are initiating some type of corrective response. Immediate correction should be the goal. At the same time, there has to be some type of assessment. "How did this happen?" Our system should be designed to make it hard for people to do the wrong thing and easy for people to do the right thing. If an error has been identified, there must be an enabling process in place so that it can be addressed. In order to fix a problem, education alone does not help. It certainly is the first step but changing your process to prevent that error from repeating itself should be hand in hand with education.

Case Study:

"We have a team experienced in mobile vaccination clinics, traveling to local offices in the community, providing vaccines, using small personal coolers to transport, storing vaccines in on-site refrigerators, using ice in plastic bags to help maintain vaccine temperatures. After reviewing the CDC Storage and Handling Toolkit, we're reconsidering other approaches. Where should we start?" The good news is, this team has a desire to vaccinate and a desire to improve!

This should be addressed with all three of our components of vaccine management in a mobile setting. 1) Equipment in this scenario is critical. Suitable vaccine transport containers or plug-in refrigerators must be used when traveling off-site. Personal coolers should never be used to transport vaccines because they are not able to maintain the required temperatures consistently. Buffered probes and digital data loggers will help assess and ensure that the temperature for vaccine storage is within the correct range and data indicating those temperatures are recorded. A simple refrigerator or environmental thermometer will not accurately reflect the temperature that the vaccine is experiencing due to the potential to fluctuate significantly with the opening and closing of the container. However, a buffered probe in glycol solution, placed in the center of the approved vaccine pack-out container, more accurately mimics the vaccine temperature rather than assessing the ambient temperature of a given environment. When trying to manage a busy off-site clinic, it is a good idea to appoint someone to set an hourly phone alarm to check the log-tag temperature and record. If it appears to be going in an upward or downward trend, this enables personnel to determine and implement a course of action quickly.

Certain scenarios may exist that in the event of an emergency, such as a power outage without a backup generator. If this occurs, clinics must quickly transport precious vaccine to another facility that has agreed to hold the vaccine under acceptable temperature storage conditions until the issue has been resolved. If these more expensive units approved for ideal vaccine transport are not available, coolers with cardboard dividers and conditioned water bottles (previously frozen and thawed to the point that the ice spins within the bottle) are used to transport in an emergency. Clinics maintaining vaccine should have written emergency plans and equipment in place before it is needed. Those plans should be exercised regularly to make sure personnel are trained, and backup facility plans are still operable. Also, best practice maintains that when transporting vaccines, it should not be drawn up in advance or transported in anything other than its original packaging. The original packaging protects it from the light, which can be detrimental and significantly helps to maintain stable temperatures. Once a vaccine is drawn into a syringe or a needle placed on a prefilled syringe, it must be protected from external contamination. More about safe injection practices and infection control is discussed in Chapter 3 of this book.

Examples of systems and processes for vaccine transport include elements such as keeping transport containers in the passenger compartment of the car and not in the trunk. Keeping vaccines out of direct sunlight and not placing containers directly on hot pavement. This may cause your equipment to work harder than needed to maintain a stable temperature, or it may not maintain it for as long a time as required or expected. Make sure staff keep transport containers closed as much as possible. Maximum transport time is going to be about eight hours or considerably less depending on the conditions and type of equipment used. Multi-dose vials (MDV) cannot be returned to the supplier if opened, nor can they be transported across state lines.

A reconstituted vaccine that is inadvertently frozen may be killed by irreversibly breaking the bond of the vaccine with the adjuvant or other vaccine components. Reconstituting live vaccines and not administering within the acceptable manufacturer window will affect the viability of the vaccine. Our intuition tells us that a vaccine which is supposed to be cold or frozen may be adversely affected by warmer temperatures. However, vaccines stored at colder than acceptable temperatures may also be harmful and destroy the vaccine altogether. In contrast, warmer than average temperatures may, over time, lead to slow degradation of the vaccine. Any time an "excursion" occurs, the vaccine must be immediately isolated to prevent use, until the manufacturer, VFC Program (if VFC vaccine), or State or local Health Department has been contacted for guidance and further direction.

Maintaining the hourly vaccine temperature log for an off-site clinic should be assigned to a responsible person, and supporting documentation should be stored at the practice even after the off-site clinic is complete. It is crucial to maintain these logs so that the integrity of the vaccines can always be verified even after they have been taken off-site and returned. Logs should be structured so they enable the required documentation. For example, if hourly temperature documentation is needed, then the log must have sufficient space for those documentation elements. The log should also have notations regarding the accepted temperature ranges for the vaccine and a place to document any corrective action that has occurred. An example of a temperature log has been included in the tools and resource section of this chapter.

In the case study, there was a reference to using "ice in a bag" to maintain the temperatures. We have to remember that ice is just frozen water, and it will return to water over time. If you elect to use something like ice in a baggie, you are putting your vaccine next to water that is unsterile and may be contaminated. If vaccines are pre-drawn into syringes and placed in a baggie with ice, the syringe may become contaminated. This would be an example of a violation of safe injection practice by pre lling and activating a syringe, which presents an opportunity to become contaminated, thus causing our patient to be at risk of harm.

Managing vaccines may seem a daunting task when combined with other functions, one may be assigned to in an office setting. A word of advice would be to not skimp on the time training takes to become proficient in this area, or the equipment involved in maintaining these important assets. Appointing an organized and diligent individual with attention to detail may also prove to be beneficial. Often a passionate "vaccine champion" is key to getting everyone on board to celebrate and respect this vital service we provide to our patients. Having the right people in the right seats on the bus can be a make or break scenario when it comes to vaccine management. We want to make sure that every patient we encounter has an equal opportunity for best practice. Best practice means safe practice. So training, testing, not being afraid to identify an error, in fact seeking an error so that you can correct it is the way we ensure patient safety.

We must remember, it may be a family member or someone important to you, receiving vaccine via this approach, whether in a drive-through in a large urban area, or employee health sites in healthcare facilities. The majority of care that occurs across the US occurs in rural settings, in small settings, in small communities. These off-site vaccine clinic plans have been created to apply to a four-hour drive through or a mobile clinic deployed in a small community, a church parking lot, a skate park, a football stadium in a large urban area, or a medical center parking area. Every process should be similar enough no matter where it is implemented or under what circumstances. The same safety components are in place in every scenario.

Local health departments often have deep roots within communities and are generally experts at immunization. Consider using this wealth of information that can be an excellent resource for any type of vaccine-related question.

Luanne Didelot MHA MSN, Ruth Carrico PhD DNP FNP-C

The focus of this chapter is on the various documentation items that facilitate patient education regarding the vaccines as well as documentation items necessary to communicate immunization across providers and healthcare settings. Vaccine Information Statements (VIS) are information sheets produced by the CDC to explain both the bene ts and the risk of a vaccine to the vaccine recipient. Federal law requires that providers give a VIS to the patient before each dose of certain vaccines. The VIS is available in about 35 different languages and is written, so those with low-literacy levels are likely to understand the contents. The federal law states that we have up to six months to begin using the newest version of a VIS. The link to the most recent VIS statements can be found on the CDC website. Information provided by the VIS should be supplemented with good patient teaching. Federal law also requires that providers report the date the patient was provided with the VIS as well as the version they were given.

If you happen to have small children and you have been to the pediatrician's office, you are very familiar with these! If you are planning a flu clinic this fall and will be offering both LAIV and inactivated flu vaccine, you will need to plan to have bother on hand as these are two distinctly different vaccines. The date located in the bottom right-hand corner of page two of the VIS would be the version that should be recorded that was provided to the patient. There is also a QR code/2D barcode in that space. If a clinic utilizes a newer electronic health record that has the capability for barcode scanner usage, clicking on the barcode will automatically document that information in an EHR. A little practical knowledge from our experience is that when you administer a vaccine to a patient, one of the most common things they are going to ask you is "what kind of side effects can I expect from the vaccine?" Point out Section 4 of the VIS and reassure them that the side effects listed are considered somewhat common or expected potential reactions to your vaccination. Such as reiterating to your patient, if it is an intramuscular injection,, "one in 15 patients are going to have a sore arm or pain at that injection site", "headache or muscle aches may be common with this vaccine",,and so forth. It may save a lot of calls to your clinic,,asking "is this normal"?" by taking the time to point out common reactions listed on the VIS statement.

Acceptable strategies to provide vaccine information statements may include having a laminated copy to present to patients while waiting for their vaccination. If a clinic is planning on sending, for example, an “online sign-up” to patients, in the event of a large scale influenza vaccine clinic, you can attach a copy of the VIS to the email, so that you know the patient actually received it and has the opportunity to go back and review if needed. However, it is always good to encourage people to take a paper copy because it also has information on the second page regarding the Vaccine Adverse Event Reporting System (VAERS). In the event the patient has a concern about a reaction, they've got the needed information in hand. If you were providing both LAIV and inactivated influenza vaccines, or including other types of vaccines at your event, consider having your copies color-coded. This allows you to quickly identify the appropriate VIS for the vaccine and helps align labels and other items to help prevent error.

If patients are presenting at a drive-through vaccination clinic, you can always ask patients to take a picture of the VIS or a QR code, so the information is available on their phone, and if they any questions, they can refer back to it. That can be a helpful strategy in addition to having multiple copies available that patients may or may not take. Patients may be reluctant to take the paper, so another alternative can be to have them take a picture of the QR code with their phone's camera. It will automatically go to the website for VIS information. Paper that gets left behind in the waiting room or wherever cannot be helpful to anyone.

The following is a case study for review: "I know that documentation is important, our EHR requires name brand of vaccine, lot number, isn't that enough? And why do these registries come into play? Why don't we hear about that? Why is it so important? And why is it important that this information is available to others? And do I want my personal information shared?"

In addressing some of those questions, the graphic on the Immunization Information System (IIS) provided in the tools and resource section of this chapter visually walks through the basics of the Immunization Information System (IIS). IIS has previously been referred to as the "State Immunization Registry," but we know it is so much more than that. It is a repository of information, and it is a wonderful planning tool. It should be the place where we gather, and we send all of our information to capture the vaccines that are administered to all people across the lifespan.

When the Immunization Information System (IIS) started taking on a life of its own, it initially focused on childhood vaccines. People are going to need vaccine records (and vaccines) up to adulthood for entering the military, applying to nursing school, dental school, medical school, joining the Peace Corps, or a wide variety of job-related requirements. We also know that some vaccines are age-appropriate and may require more than one dose.

To ensure accuracy, vaccination series completion, appropriateness of spacing, and other essential vaccination considerations, we must have a reliable way of documenting and communicating across providers and systems. We are gaining a greater appreciation for how vital access to our immunization records has become. It enables accurate immunization and preventing inappropriate spacing, missed doses, and promotes adherence to the CDC in the ACIP guidelines at all stages of life.

A federal IIS did not come to fruition many years ago since states had unique and varied jurisdictional needs. For that reason, individual states developed their own State Immunization Registries. They may look a bit different but operate mainly based upon the same principles. Some states have registries that look strikingly similar, which is because they are developed and/or managed by the same vendor. That would seem to make it plausible that in the future, they have the potential to become interoperable.

In terms of confidentiality of the IIS, entering immunizations into the registry is exempt from the Privacy Rule because this is considered a public health activity. Only physicians, nurse practitioners, and physician assistant providers, pharmacists, school nurses and other healthcare workers, have access to the information. Patients can have access to their own records as well. You can also request individual access to get your child's record. Patients can opt-out of the IIS by contacting their state. However, very few patients are choosing to exercise that option.

Federal law requires documentation following immunization to include: the name of the vaccine manufacturer, the brand name of the vaccine, lot number, expiration date, date administered, the name, address, title, of the healthcare provider administering the vaccine. The law does not require that we obtain consent to give immunization. It merely requires that we are going to document that we answered questions, gave the patient the appropriate VIS, and the date we provided that to the patient. Therefore, a written consent form for vaccination is not required. You may elect to use a consent form for a drive-through immunization as a means of verifying patients who may not already be part of your practice and enabling contact with them. This may be important to consider in the unlikely event there is a vaccine recall, injection practice error, or some other need to reach those you vaccinated.

There are still some practices utilizing paper medical records, but for the most part, providers are using some sort of Electronic Health Record (EHR). Many years ago, we believed the advent of the EHR to be the panacea for providers and their patients. Digitizing medical records was going to save time, improve care for patients by not duplicating services, and save money. The unintended consequence soon became evident that providers were utilizing and contributing to "silos of information". The issue is that these "silos" are not "talking" or sharing information. The IIS is the exception to that general scenario. Providers or office staff may not be constantly aware. Still, their electronic health record, in many instances, is auto-populating immunizations they administer into the state registry, which is a tremendous achievement! It is an information exchange. Sometimes it is unidirectional, meaning a provider enters information into their electronic health record in the immunization table, and it transmits to the state registry. Some IIS can work vice versa (bi-directional), meaning the state IIS could auto-populate a health system's EHR, depending on how robust an EHR system is and its proprietary coding.

We have alluded a bit into the many ways in which data entry into the IIS can occur, including manual entry (typing of the vaccine information directly into the IIS, which does not sound very appealing! A barcode scanner is another method that may be available, depending upon the sophistication level of the EHR. With the click of a scanner on the vaccine's 2D or linear barcode, this information can be instantly uploaded into the patient's immunization record. Like retail products, there is a lot of data stored in barcodes that does the work for you. A provider's electronic medical record can populate the state registry in that manner. It may be worth a discussion with your facility information technology department to determine existing capabilities that will be beneficial during a drive-through vaccination event.

Why would you want to document vaccine information? We know that federal law requires us to do so, but besides that, it simplifies record keeping and reduces chances for unnecessary doses. One unique feature is the evaluation and forecasting tool. If a parent is sending their child to summer camp and they need proof of immunization, the state registry has an option to print the official record with a state seal. It is straightforward to retrieve that information and print it for those purposes. A reminder recall is also an attractive feature for providers and families. Often during the middle and high school years, busy families may be a bit less diligent with the cycle of annual well-child visits that they were in during the infant and toddler years. In middle school, adolescents are due to begin the recommended HPV series. Follow-up with subsequent doses can fall by the wayside if we do not see the adolescent for a while, until they need something else from us. Assume the patient returns after a hiatus, we are well aware, based on the IIS, that they may be overdue for the

HPV vaccination in the series.

It is critical that when we have patients coming to a drive-through for any vaccine, we fulfill our responsibility in getting the information into the state registry. If a child requires a second dose, this registry will enable the parent and/or provider to know what vaccine was administered when, and what is currently due. Prevention of missed or unneeded doses is vitally important. We should not rely on patient's verbal reports that they had their influenza, pneumonia, or shingles vaccines, for example, as those with experience know, that can be problematic and involve unreliable information.

The number of patients with vaccines in the IIS decreases dramatically with age. Due to the length of time IIS has been in use and the apparent need for the early focus on children via state mandates would explain the differences. Another motivating reason to utilize IIS is the mobile nature of our society. It is estimated by the CDC that 20% of children over the age of two have already been to more than one medical provider. The American Community Survey indicates that individuals move an estimated 11 times during their lifetime. Newborns receive their first Hepatitis B vaccine while hospitalized. Children up to 24 months are receiving the bulk of their pediatric vaccinations, "kindergarten shots" follow, and by the time the child turns eleven, meningococcal and T-dap may be needed to meet the state school requirement. College preparation generally includes meningococcal as well. Young adults in their 20's may be childbearing years for a lot of folks, needing T-dap again, MMR, or other vaccinations. Starting in our 50's, we are recommended to receive the shingles vaccine, and 65 and older are receiving pneumococcal. This is a significant illustration of the importance of IIS.

The American Immunization Registry Association (AIRA) is an organization focused on pulling these individual state registries together and pushing them forward, to elevate the role and the importance of using the infrastructure currently in place. With the anticipation of COVID-19 vaccines on the horizon, we can indeed surmise the impact that IIS will have going forward. As COVID-19 has compelled us to find alternative ways to provide vaccinations (e.g., drive-through clinics) and office visits via telemedicine. Surely the prospect of having multiple COVID-19 vaccines on the market with different schedules and dosing will further elevate the mission and acknowledgment of the essential nature of IIS. The AIRA continues to accelerate the on boarding of providers and health systems and addressing barriers to the process of preparing for the future wave of challenges.

Information about every patient receiving immunization is critical, and we have the opportunity to prevent disease and promote health. So, regardless of where we provide vaccines, we must think about and remember “patient first”. The patient is the center of what we are doing. They are the beacon that is guiding us in all of our actions. Ensuring that we enable them to receive best-practice care requires documentation and active use of the immunization registries. IIS is an ideal way to do that. There are challenges, and it can be time-consuming, and some are easier than others. But you know, a way to change that is not just ignoring it. Instead, we need to actively work and advocate for the patient to make those types of changes. But in the interim, making sure that we have documentation is essential for their care. Whether you are providing influenza vaccine alone or using drive-through as an opportunity to provide a way for the public to ‘catch up’ on missed vaccines, use of the IIS is essential in ensuring best practice care for vaccine-preventable diseases.

CHAPTER 7

DRIVE-THROUGH VACCINATION: EMERGENCY RESPONSE IN A DRIVE-THROUGH VACCINATION EVENT

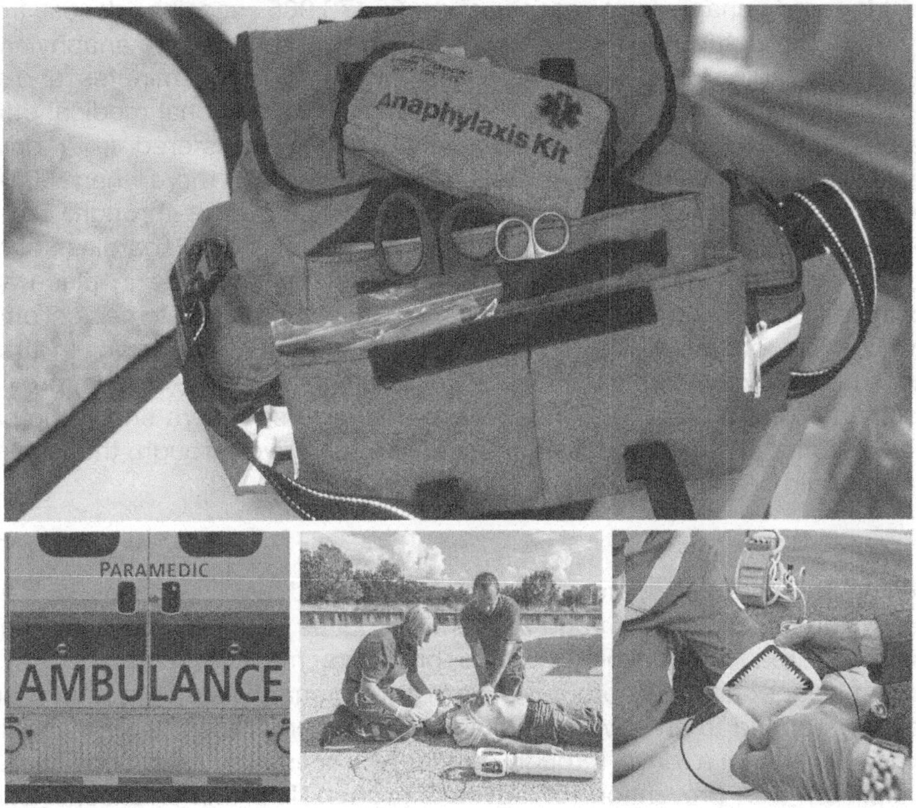

Dawn Balcom DNP FNP-C, Ruth Carrico PhD DNP FNP-C

Severe adverse vaccine reactions administered in any setting are rare. However, rapid recognition and immediate treatment are required to prevent possible advancement of respiratory distress or cardiovascular collapse. The Food and Drug Administration (FDA) Vaccine Adverse Event Reporting System (VAERS) reports that approximately 30,000 VAERS reports are filed yearly, and 85-90% of the accounts describe mild side effects such as fever, arm soreness, and crying or mild irritability. More severe reactions are rare. The Journal of Allergy and Clinical Immunology reported 33 confirmed vaccine-triggered anaphylaxis cases after 25,173,965 vaccine doses from January 2009 through 2011 [1]. This is equivalent to a rate of 1.31 anaphylactic events per one million doses. Symptom onset was within 30 minutes and 24 hours. An adverse reaction to a vaccine provided in a traditional medical office is a rare event, and it is also a rare event when administered in a drive-through process. Over fifteen years, from 1995-2010, more than 50,000 vaccines were administered in Louisville, Kentucky, via a drive-through. During this time, there were no reported vaccine adverse events [2]. Regardless of the rarity of an event, measures that ensure patient safety must be in place and must be able to be implemented. The provision of vaccination in a medical office or pharmacy includes an ability to respond to an emergent condition. In those settings, emergency interventions such as an ability to adequate screen, provide emergency medication, and communicate with first responders should be part of routine practice. When a vaccine is provided via a drive-through, those same measures should be in place, so safe care is provided.

Emergency preparedness for managing an adverse event, or any emergency, during a drive-through event, requires having an emergency response plan readily available. Vaccine providers must be competent with recognizing signs and symptoms of an acute anaphylactic reaction and confident to respond to an adverse event rapidly. When preparing for managing an adverse event in a drive-through setting, process development should focus first on the prevention of adverse events. The Immunization Action Coalition (IAC) has developed screening checklists to aid in identifying possible contraindications to vaccine administration [3]. Vaccine providers must also be knowledgeable of common vaccine ingredients that may trigger an allergic event. The CDC has developed a list of the type of ingredients found in vaccines that should be readily accessible on-site for the vaccine providers to reference [4]. Screening handout examples and the CDC list of vaccine ingredients are included in the tools and resource section of this chapter.

Syncope, although uncommon, can occur during or after a vaccine has been administered. Providing a little extra time with anxious participants can reduce fear and reduce the risk of syncope. Once fear or hesitance is recognized by the vaccine provider, there are several techniques to help reduce anxiety and reassure the participant. Calmly and unhurriedly speak to the participant. If they share something specific that is making them feel uneasy, acknowledge that you hear them but reassure that you will help them through the process. Ask the participant a question that requires more than a yes or no answer. For example, ask, "what are you going to have for lunch today?" Advise the participant to concentrate on taking slow deep breaths, all the way down into their belly, or to turn the radio and find a song or station they enjoy. If unable to calm the anxious participant in a reasonable time frame, ask them to either proceed forward to a designated area to park the vehicle. Plan to have an additional vaccine provider available to engage with anxious vaccine recipients. The participant can always make the personal decision to drive away. If the patient feels "faint", have the patient recline their seat back or lie flat and loosen any tight clothes. Plan to keep a few damp, cold towels on-site to apply to the face and neck and stay and observe until the individual feels they have fully recovered [5]. If loss of consciousness occurs, check to determine if an injury is present before attempting to move them. Place them flat on their back with feet elevated. Call 911 if they do not recover immediately.

In the event of an anaphylactic reaction, which is defined by the International Consensus on Anaphylaxis as "a serious, generalized or systemic, allergic or hypersensitivity reaction that can be life-threatening or fatal", the drive-through emergency response plan should be activated. Vaccine providers must quickly recognize the signs/symptoms of an anaphylactic reaction and immediately call 911 for assistance. Each team member should know their role in the event of an emergency. All vaccination providers should be certi ed in cardiopulmonary resuscitation.

The following is a general review of anaphylaxis presentation and intervention. Anaphylaxis is a systemic reaction that produces the following signs and symptoms:

- Skin and mucosal symptoms such as generalized hives, itching or ushing
- Swelling of lips, face, throat, or eye
- Respiratory symptoms such as stridor, shortness of breath, wheezing or cough, nasal congestion
- A change in voice
- A sensation of throat closing
- Gastrointestinal symptoms such as nausea, vomiting, diarrhea, cramping abdominal pain

- Cardiovascular symptoms such as collapse, dizziness, tachycardia, hypotension

If the participant exhibits respiratory or cardiovascular symptoms or other signs or symptoms of anaphylaxis, immediate intramuscular Epinephrine is the first-line treatment of choice.

- Epinephrine 1 mg/ml aqueous solution (1:1000 dilution) in prefilled autoinjector or prefilled syringe (various doses), prepackaged syringes, vials, or ampules.

The Immunization Action Coalition recommends at least three doses should be available on-site, dosages as appropriate for the patient population.

Other medications to have available are Diphenhydramine and Hydroxyzine. These medications are given to relieve itching and hives only; they DO NOT relieve upper or lower airway obstruction, hypotension, or shock.

- Diphenhydramine (e.g., Benadryl) oral, 12.5mg/5ml Liquid; 25 or 50 mg tablets
- Hydroxyzine (e.g., Atarax, Vistaril) oral, 10mg/5ml; 10 or 25 mg tablets

After administering Epinephrine to the patient, and while awaiting the arrival of EMS to arrive, it is essential to listen to the individual and follow their lead. For example, if the person verbalizes the need to sit upright or stand up to breathe, do not force them to lie down. If and when the person becomes hypotensive, place them in a recumbent position with the legs elevated. Maintain the airway, provide oxygen if available, monitor vital signs, and repeat Epinephrine as needed. After the patient is stabilized, they should be transported by EMS to an emergency facility for additional monitoring. Anaphylaxis can reoccur even after the person has begun to recover.

During the preparation phase for a drive-through event, contact your local emergency service director to inquire about the provision of an ambulance unit to stay on-site or close by during the event. It is also beneficial to contact the local 911 call center and share information regarding the drive-through event. Provide the dispatcher specific details on the who, what, where, when, and why of the event. Consider packing a colorful flag or cloth that you can use as a means of identifying your location. Provide your team members with specific information to relay to 911 dispatch in the event of an emergency. A script with this information could be sent via text to each team member to use as a reference in the event of an emergency.

A script with this information could be texted to each team member to use as a reference in the event of an emergency. The more details you can provide to the dispatcher regarding your exact location will reduce the estimated time of arrival of an ambulance to your site. One example of a script might be: "My name is John Doe. I am with a 50-year-old man who is having a severe anaphylactic reaction to a vaccine. We are located at Green St. Church. The address here is 1678 Longstay Place. It is close to (provide a landmark). We are in room 3A in the basement of the church. Please have the ambulance drive to the back of the building and enter into the doors located on the right side of the back of the church. We will have someone waiting outside the door holding up a red towel to help you find our location".

Stay calm for the benefit of the person you are assisting. Remember, when an emergency arises, minutes seem like forever!

The Immunization Action Coalition has developed standing orders for emergency preparedness in a community setting that is comprehensive and provides detailed guidance through the event.

The standing order provides advice for required medications, equipment needed, and medication dosing per weight and age. Below is an example of the Epinephrine dosing guide, which can be laminated and placed in the emergency bag with emergency drugs. This guide provides quick access for Epinephrine dosing for infants, children, and teens.

The Immunization Action Coalition standing orders are included in the tools and resource section of this chapter, and they can also be accessed at the following links:

https://www.immunize.org/catg.d/p3082.pdf (Adults)
https://www.immunize.org/catg.d/p3082a.pdf (Children & Teens)

First-Line Treatment: Epinephrine					**Epinephrine Dose**	
		Age group	Range of weight (lb)	Range of weight (kg)*	1.0 mg/ml aqueous solution (1:1000 dilution); intramuscular. Minimum dose 0.05 mL	Epinephrine autoinjector of prefilled syringe (0.1mg, 0.15 mg, 0.3 mg
Recommended dose is 0.01 mg/kg body weight up to 0.5 mg maximum dose.	Infants and Children	1-6 months	9-19 lb	4-8.5 kg	0.05 mL (or mg)	Off Label
		7-36 months	20-32 lb^	9-14.5 kg^	0.1 mL (or mg)	0.1 mg
		37-59 months	33-39 lb	15-17.5 kg	0.15 mL (or mg)	0.15 mg/dose
		5-7 years	40-56 lb	18-25.5 kg	0.2-0.25 mL (or mg)	0.15 mg/dose
		8-10 years	57-76 lb	26-34.5 kg	0.25-0.3 mL (or mg)	0.15 mg or 0.3 mg/dose
May be repeated every 5-15 minutes (or sooner) up to 3 times while waiting for EMS to arrive.	Teens	11-12 years	77-99 lb	35-45 kg	0.35-0.4 mL (or mg)	0.3 mg/dose
		13 years & older	100+ lb	46+ kg	0.5 mL (or mg) - maximum dose	0.3 mg/dose
NOTE: If bodyweight is known, then dosing by weight is preferred. If weight is not known or not readily available, dosing by age is appropriate				*Rounded weight at the 50th percentile for each age range ^ 0.1 mg autoinjector is licensed for use in 7.5-14 kg infants and children		

Any adverse event that occurs after administering a vaccine must be reported to VAERS. If you are uncertain if the adverse event was caused by the vaccine, complete the VAERS report. The reports are signals that alert scientists of possible cause-and-effect relationships that need to be investigated.

When reviewing steps in identifying contraindications to individual vaccines, preparing to answer questions from recipients regarding vaccine components, and ensuring that your team has visual resources at their fingertips in the event emergency intervention is needed, an excellent reference is the CDC Pink Book. This book contains information for routine vaccines and a comprehensive set of appendices that provide a full array of resources useful for all settings and all personnel involved in immunization procedures. The Pink Book is in hard copy as well as electronic and can be accessed at https://www.cdc.gov/vaccines/pubs/pinkbook/index.html. Contemporary ideas to provide preventive vaccines to the community are necessary now more than ever. The COVID-19 pandemic has significantly reduced routine vaccination rates, so alternative ways of providing immunization to individuals of all ages while enabling social distancing and other infection control measures can be of tremendous value to communities of all sizes.

Drive-through events are one alternative to provide vaccines safely and efficiently. Adverse events in any setting are rare. However, planning and preparedness for managing a severe adverse event can be lifesaving. Please take the time to review the tools and resources https://www.cdc.gov/vaccines/hcp/acip-recs/general-recs/adverse-reactions.pdf

References

1. McNeil MM, Weintraub ES, Duffy J, Sukumaran L, Jacobsen SJ, Klein NP, et al. Risk of anaphylaxis after vaccination in children and adults. J Allergy Clin Immunol. 2016 Mar;137(3):868–78. https://doi.org/10.1016/j.jaci.2015.07.048 PMID:26452420
2. Carrico RM, FSHEA C, McKinney WP, Nicholas Adam Watson JD, Wiemken T, Myers J. Drive-thru influenza immunization: fifteen years of experience. Journal of Emergency Management. 2012 May 1;10(3):228-32.
3. Handouts: Topic Index. (n.d.). Retrieved August 18, 2020, from https://www.immunize.org/handouts/screening-vaccines.asp
4. Vaccines: Vac-Gen/Additives in Vaccines Fact Sheet. (2020). Retrieved August 18, 2020, from https://www.cdc.gov/vaccines/vac-gen/additives.htm
5. Immunization Action Coalition (IAC): Vaccine Information for Health Care Professionals. (n.d.). Retrieved August 19, 2020, from https://immunize.org/
6. Vaccine Adverse Event Reporting System (VAERS) | Monitoring | Ensuring Safety | Vaccine Safety | CDC. (2020). Retrieved August 18, 2020, from https://www.cdc.gov/vaccinesafety/en
7. Dreskin SC, Halsey NA, Kelso JM, Wood RA, Hummell DS, Edwards KM, et al. International Consensus (ICON): allergic reactions to vaccines. World Allergy Organ J. 2016 Sep;9(1):32. Available from: https://pubmed.ncbi.nlm.nih.gov/27679682/ https://doi.org/10.1186/s40413-016-0120-5 PMID:27679682
8. Safety Information by Vaccine | CDC. (2020). Retrieved August 18, 2020, from https://www.cdc.gov/vaccinesafety/
9. CDC. Vaccine Adverse Reactions. (2020). Retrieved August 16, 2020, from https://www.cdc.gov/vaccines/hcp/acip-recs/general-recs/adverse-reactions.pdf

CHAPTER 8

DRIVE-THROUGH VACCINATION: RIGHT-SIZING A DRIVE-THROUGH VACCINATION EVENT FOR COMMUNITY NEEDS

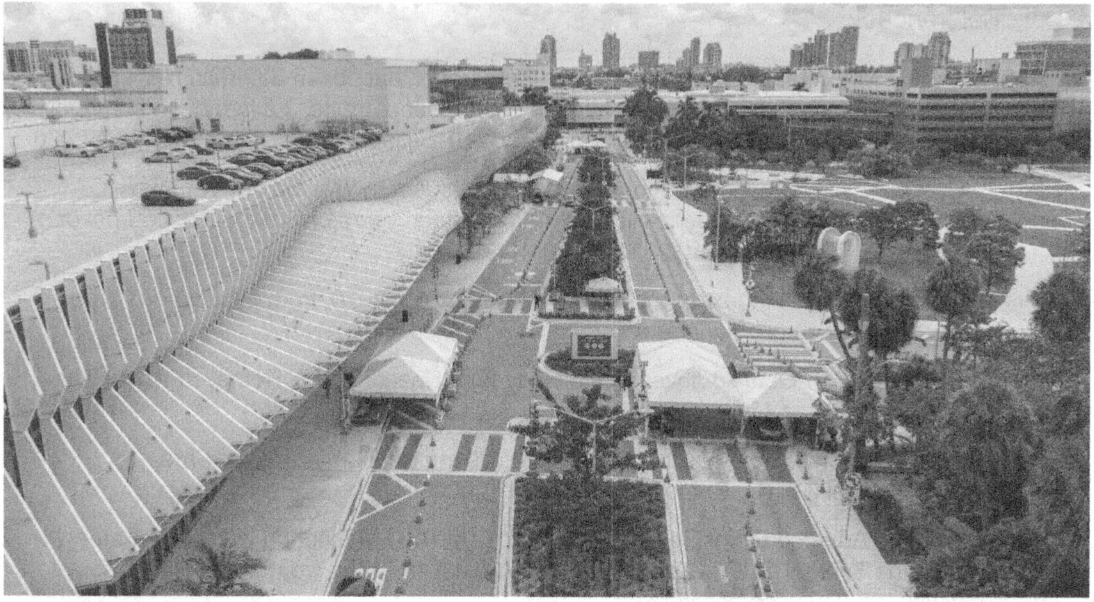

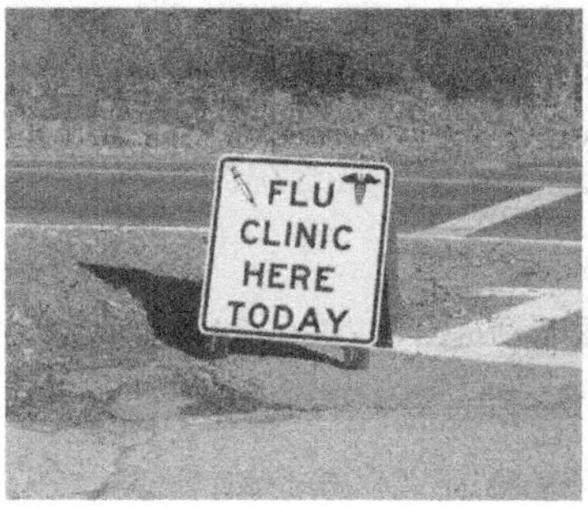

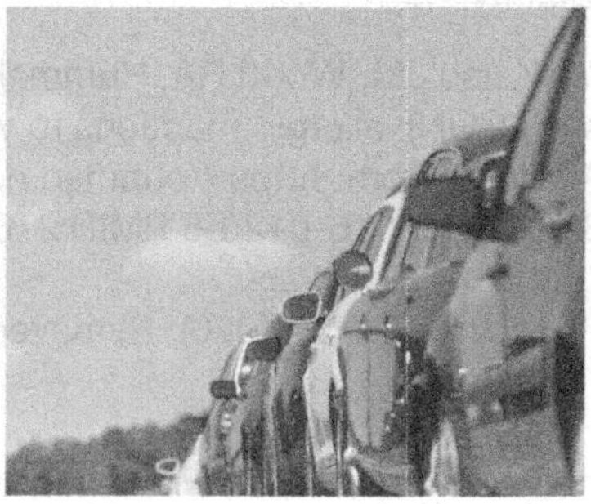

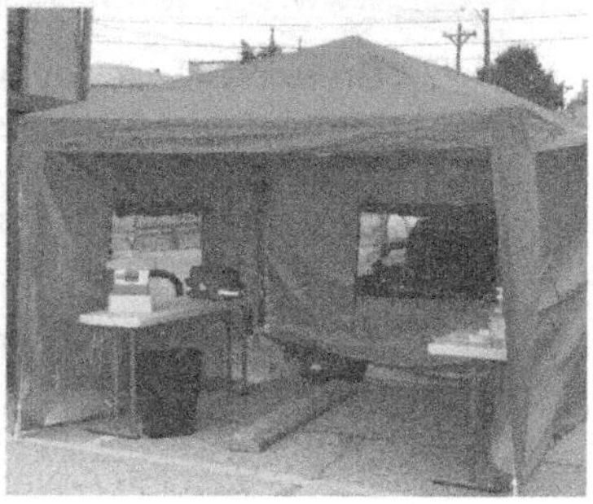

Dennis Sullivan BA, EMT-P, CHMM, CEM, Ruth Carrico PhD DNP FNP-C

Community needs for vaccination will vary due to several factors, with accessibility and availability of vaccines being primary drivers. A large immunization event is most likely to be beneficial when addressing an out-of-the-ordinary situation such as the introduction of a new vaccine, catch-up vaccinations for school settings, limited availability, or late release of an anticipated vaccine, or a community emergency. These circumstances may require that many doses of vaccine be administered in a short time period resulting in mass immunization situations. Regardless of the size of the community, the implementation of a vaccination event designed to provide a majority of the population with vaccine access will require the work of a multidisciplinary team. Fortunately, the team components are similar despite the size of the event. The primary difference is the scale.

When planning a large community event, several public health tools have been developed for such a purpose. The bio-terrorism readiness initiatives in the early part of this century served as the platform for responses generated in anticipation of an avian influenza H5N1 outbreak. They used as part of the national response to H1N1 influenza in 2009. As described in Chapter 1, planning begins with gathering the multidisciplinary team. With large events, it is critical to collaborate with local public health and other city officials to engage the level of resources that may be outside the scope of many healthcare settings. These include city traffic control around the venue area, more extensive scale communications, venue identification and selection, and access to set-up supplies and equipment for the site. NACCHO published an excellent tool that outlines large scale immunization events within the context of public health Points of Dispensing operations in 2010. This document was based upon the Louisville mass immunization experiences and is included in the tools and resource section of this chapter. Its content remains relevant to planning and conducting large scale vaccination events.

Another essential tool for large scale immunization programs is the Federal Emergency Management Agency (FEMA) National Incident Command System (NIMS). This federal approach provides a consistent template that can enable partners across multiple sectors to work together. NIMS can be used to guide structural strategies and personnel organization regardless of the situation, size, or complexity of the event. The organization process enables a command structure that is familiar to public health, emergency planners, city services, but may be foreign to many frontline workers in healthcare. The biggest challenge to healthcare personnel is the transition to a command and control management structure. This differs significantly from the teamwork that is the staple of healthcare environments where individuals are encouraged to work collaboratively and cross-departmentally. Transitioning from one management approach to the other requires training to ensure that assigned roles and tasks are completed consistently and reliably. The incident command structure, an integral NIMS component, is shown in the figure below and is helpful for planners considering drive-through vaccination events regardless of the size.

FEMA Incident Command Structure

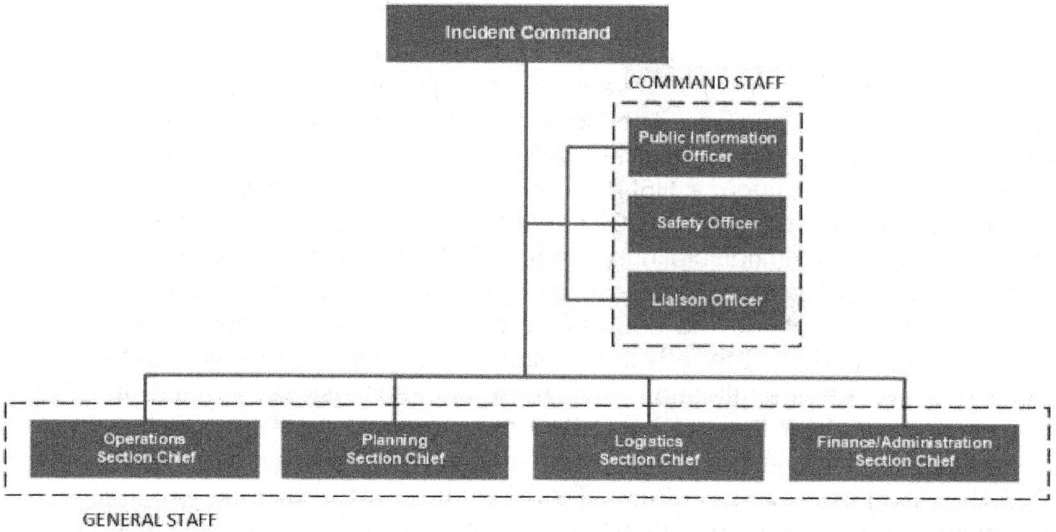

https://www.fema.gov/sites/default/les/2020-07/fema_nims_doctrine-2017.pdf

A large event, regardless of the site location, will impact local traffic, so understanding the existing traffic patterns as well as the potential impact is essential for planning. One approach is to engage individuals with expertise in industrial engineering. These specialists have been responsible for developing processes used by UPS, Amazon, and other multinational companies, so they are experts in understanding systems and improving processes. For the H1N1 immunization event in Louisville in 2009, engineers helped evaluate the throughput by measuring the time spent at each designated station (e.g., greeting, consent, vaccine administration) and the time between those stations. This helped identify the most likely locations for the delay and the targets for additional improvement attention. Developing of simulations can help bring a visual element to the discussion and enable a clear picture of the process and potential solutions. Examples of documents designed for simulation are included in the tools and resource section of this chapter.

For smaller community events, or those involving single medical practices, the same planning approaches are beneficial. The numbers of personnel needed to handle the event may not be the same, but the steps in the planning approach are similar. Relationships are vital in organizing events that require multiple partners, and this is often a specialty in smaller communities. A rural community may elect to have a vaccination event in a public area familiar to the community, such as a local park or church. The location must be screened to ensure accessibility, as well as the availability of telephone service in the event local first responder communication, is needed. Rustic areas such as parks may lack easy access to electricity, water, and toilet facilities that are necessities for a drive-through immunization event. The entire planning team should consider a complete evaluation of a venue and a vaccination process.

Marketing and communication is an important consideration regardless of the event size. Processes that help ensure there is adequate knowledge of the event among community members is critical, especially among those who may have less than adequate communication channels or input. For large events, adding communication tools that help with traffic directions can be particularly important. Use of local community radio stations with scripted messages or recordings, use of over-the-road highway signs, or portable roadside signs are examples of these resources that may be available through local emergency planning or state departments of transportation. Marketing specialists can help make sure important information is also included in print media such as the local newspaper, community newsletters, and church bulletins. Information such as event location and times of operation, as well as downloadable forms such as consent documents and VIS, are examples of what should be included in those communications.

Finances are a crucial element of a drive-through event, and this is evidenced by the need to have financial management competence as part of the planning team. Funding and available financial support may be the deciding factor as to the size and location of a drive-through event. Record keeping and real-time documentation of expenses are needed. Evaluation of the existing capital and anticipated revenue to cover all associated costs are financial components that must be planned for, and in place as planning and implementation activities begin. Finance documents should include rental items, venue rental, reusable items such as vaccine refrigerators for transport, vaccines, consumable supplies, personnel, and any additional insurance needed for the event.

Rental items may include tents and stabilizing weights, communication devices, signage, generators, electricity cables, and cords, heaters, tables, coolers for staff drinking water or other fluids, rolling carts, traffic cones, and small transport vehicles. Items and quantities depend upon the size of the event. Venue rental may include the day of the event as well as an additional day for setting up and tear down. Contracts should clearly outline what is provided and any restrictions, including other insurance requirements. Some reusable items not currently available in the clinic may need to be purchased for a drive-through event. These include vaccine refrigerators for transport, digital thermometers, open-top containers that help to separate different types of vaccines, rolling hand carts for easy movement of items, and small printers or copy machines if clerical or insurance responsibilities will be done at the drive-through event. Vaccine costs are likely to be the most considerable portion of the expenses, and often terms of payment are 90-120 days after receipt. If this is not already in place, discussing with the vaccine company/companies before delivery is advisable. Also, the companies may have an early payment discount of several percent in the event you can take advantage of it. Check on return options in the event there are vaccines unused at the end of the season. Consumable supplies include those items used for vaccination, hand caddies or carriers to maintain vaccination supplies for movement to cars, personal protective equipment, hand hygiene products, emergency response medication and kit, surface disinfectant wipes, trash receptacles, food and drink items for personnel, paper copies and lamination, disposable signs, pens, copy paper, and other consumable clerical items. Personnel costs are essential to outline at the planning phase, so you have the right people doing the right jobs, and you are accounting for the costs of their work efforts. Personnel include all members of the drive-through team, security personnel, management, and licensed provider oversight. Establishing spreadsheets with all costs, actual and projected, should begin early in the planning process.

An aspect of financial management of the drive-through vaccination event may involve the use of patient's private insurance, Medicaid, or Medicare. The complexities of insurance submission and billing are beyond the intent of this book but should be part of planning consideration. As an aid for this planning, a billing and coding manual made available by Sanofi Pasteur is included in the tools and resource section of this chapter. If the decision involves acceptance of cash/check/credit card payment, then the provision of a receipt or other information necessary for the recipient to submit the charge for insurance reimbursement should be provided at the drive-through event. Individuals coming through the event should also be provided information regarding how they should follow up regarding those claims.

There should be an opportunity to debrief with all personnel at the end of the event to use the experience as a learning opportunity and a celebration of success. A report should be developed outlining the activities involved in planning and implementation as well as a detailed financial report. This report will be of particular importance in recognizing opportunities for cost reduction and resource stewardship for the next events. With the utility and success of drive-through events for immunization as well as other healthcare activities and interventions, the lessons learned will be necessary for future activities, including how we can continue to improve immunization access to cover the entire community.

CHAPTER 9

DRIVE-THROUGH VACCINATION: BRINGING IT ALL TOGETHER FOR AN INCLUSIVE DRIVE-THROUGH VACCINATION EFFORT

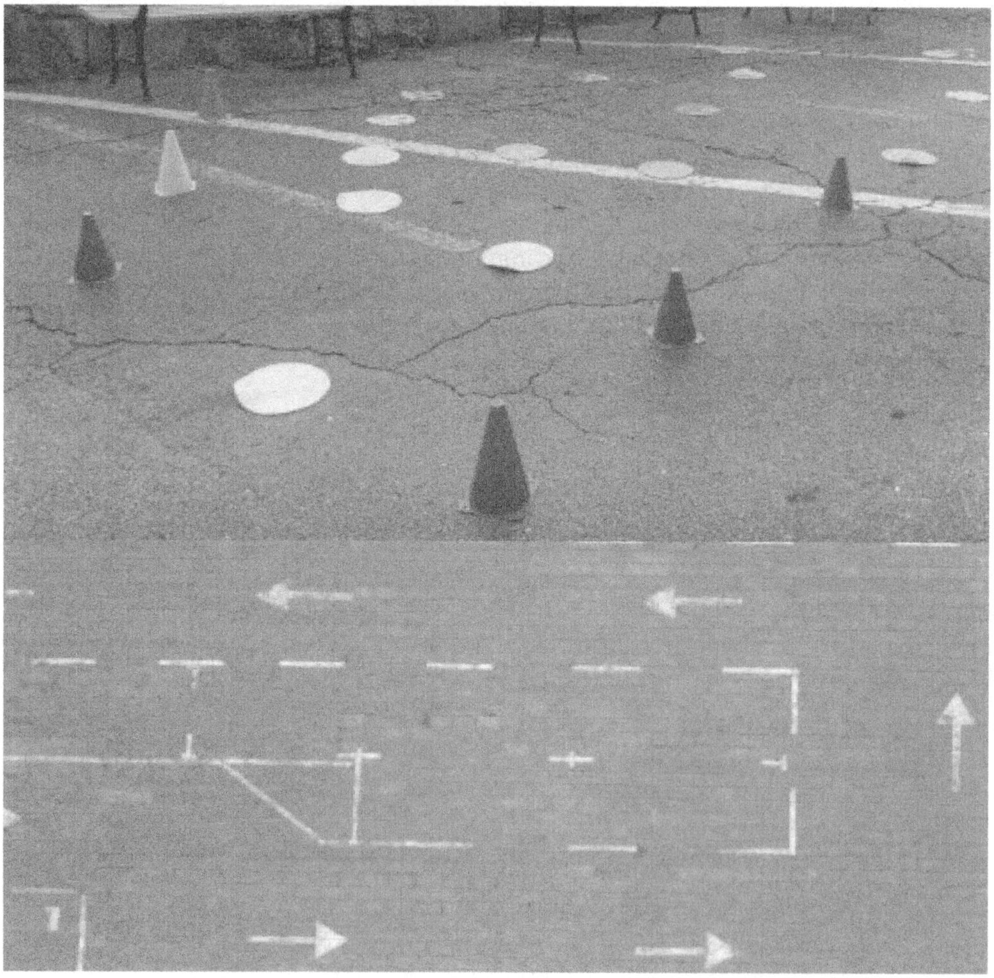

Ruth Carrico PhD DNP FNP-C

The previous chapters have reviewed the major planning elements essential in organizing a drive-through vaccination event. Each chapter has provided information along with tools and resources that can assist in efforts to enable the availability of vaccines and access to the event. Although the focus has been on drive-through, which by name suggests that the availability of a vehicle is the only way to participate, the drive-through process can be used in a variety of ways. This becomes important for community consideration as the public health importance of immunization is a right and, as such, must be provided to all members of society as all members of society benefit.

Drive-through processes can be used in areas of the community where access to a car may or may not exist. Planners should consider the use of the process in areas where individuals may carpool or when city buses can bring them together. Churches, shopping centers, and community centers are examples of those sites. The same components of social distancing and infection control can be implemented, regardless of the setting. The key is the creativity and engagement of community members able to pull populations together and encourage vaccination. Poverty is a driving force in chronic and communicable diseases. Therefore, it is incumbent upon members in a civilized society to confront that barrier to widespread public health and take the necessary steps. The use of a drive-through process for vaccination can be a valuable tool in this effort.

As preparations move forward for large scale, mass community immunization as a countermeasure against COVID-19, the ability to conceptualize an event capable of vaccinating the majority of a community population can follow the formulas outlined in this book. Additional activities for such an event include the following planning considerations:

- Identifying an adequate venue capable of handling the anticipated traffic is a first step in the planning process. If there is the ability to engage industrial engineers to help design the process, this may help ensure appropriate throughput that can handle the volume of vehicles that are anticipated.
- An adequate venue should also be capable of accepting public transportation to ensure that community members without individual vehicles can receive a vaccination.
- If more than one dose of the vaccine is required, venue planning should include a second drive-through date within the required time frame for dose spacing.

- Providing additional consent documents and an adequate explanation of the vaccine may be required. If a vaccine is released under an FDA emergency use authorization, a more extensive consent document outlining elements such as known adverse events and clinical trials results are part of ethical practice. This information enables community members to make informed decisions as they weigh the risks and benefits of the vaccine against the risks of the targeted disease.

- Storage capabilities for the many doses of vaccine available for administration, it is likely that vaccines may need to be centrally stored to monitor access and storage conditions. If routine refrigerated or frozen conditions are required, existing storage capabilities in a health department or large pharmacy may be sufficient. If, however, additional conditions are required, such as ultra-low freezing temperatures (e.g., -70°C), it is critical to investigate where those storage conditions are available. Commercial grade freezers will be unable to reach and maintain those ultra-low temperatures, so local research universities are one source to consider.

- A large workforce competent to handle and administer vaccines can be achieved by working with local schools of nursing, the local medical society, and pharmacies. Vaccines may be delivered in multi-dose vials without a preservative. Therefore, personnel must have firm practice competence in infection control and safe injection practices. If diluents are used, personnel must be trained on the additional complexities required for vaccines that may require additional handling. Personnel must also be capable of monitoring time-dependent stability (e.g., a vaccine must be administered within a speci ed period after the vial is first accessed) and ensure each administered dose has been maintained under correct conditions. Training is crucial and must be standardized to the extent possible.

- Supply levels must be available to address vaccine administration needs. Ample supplies of needles, syringes, alcohol swabs, Band-Aids, and emergency response medication must be readily available and remain stored under suitable conditions.

- A database capable of providing information enabling tracking of vaccine recipients is vital. This is important to monitor for adverse events and enable receipt of followup dose(s) of vaccine if needed. The ability to protect the personal information of the recipient as well as report information necessary to monitor vaccine safety must be considered at the time the database is developed. Ensuring data maintenance and integrity will be a challenge, so creating an initial paper process might be an important consideration even though it seems antiquated.

- Advanced scheduling may be used, but planners should be aware that there may be a concern within the public that they may not be able to receive the vaccine if they wait for their turn. Therefore, planners should be prepared to expect large numbers of vehicles to report to the vaccination site well before the scheduled hours of operation.

For success, the community must come together with a focus on ensuring access to vaccine for as many as possible. Planning must have a strategy for identifying those at highest risk and devoting e orts to making their access to vaccine a reality. The willingness to work together for the good of all represents the most outstanding achievement of society. Making this happen during a pandemic requires commitment from all.

VIDEO SERIES

- LOGISTICS & CLINIC SET-UP
- STAFF & TRANING
- INFECTION CONTROL & SAFE INJECTION PRACTICES
- VACCINE & SUPPLY INVENTORY MANAGEMENT
- VACCINE STORAGE, TRANSPORT & TEMPERATURE MONITORING
- PATIENT EDUCATION, DOCUMENTATION, VIS & EMERGENCY RESPONSE IN A DRIVE-THROUGH VACCINATION EVENT
- RIGHT-SIZING A DRIVE-THROUGH VACCINATION EVENT FOR COMMUNITY NEEDS
- BRINGING IT ALL TOGETHER FOR AN INCLUSIVE DRIVE-THROUGH EFFORT

Made in the USA
Monee, IL
08 November 2026

67969857R00046